WALLABY

WOK
YOUR WAY
SKINNY!

ANNETTE ANNECHILD

Food Consultant: Skip Skwarek

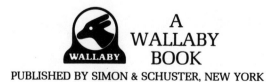

A
WALLABY
BOOK
PUBLISHED BY SIMON & SCHUSTER, NEW YORK

WALLABY and colophon are registered trademarks of Simon & Schuster
First Wallaby Books printing October 1982
7   9   10   8   6
Manufactured in the United States of America
Printed and bound by Maple-Vail Book Manufacturing Group
ISBN: 0-671-42691-5

This book is humbly dedicated
to my beloved Gurudev,

who taught me that
the true weight is the weight
of the ego.

With special thanks to:

Jimmy Glenn
Steven Joseph
Skip Skwarek
Linda Chambers
Russell Bennett
My Parents, Anne and Frank Viscardi
Laura Bialosky
Ed and Eileen Friedman
John Boswell
Charles Stetler, Jon Elliot, Lynda West
Gene Brissie
The Tint Family
Dr. Randolph Meltzer
Jean and John Holdampf
Arnie Shapiro and my Fire Island family
And to Sahm, Cathy and Jerry Laks, wherever they are . . .

*Your hard work and soft love are the essential
ingredients in my recipe for successful books
and happy living.*

CONTENTS

7 LUNCH ON THE GO | 71

8 DYNAMITE DINNERS | 83

9 SAVORY SOUPS | 121

10 DAZZLING DESSERTS | 137

11 MAKING THIS WORK FOR YOU | 151

1

FEELING FAT

I'd never trust a diet book written by somebody who had never been fat. You have to have been there to know.

Well, I've been there and I know—the frustration, the obsession, the sense of failure, the self-hatred. Fat is a state of mind as well as body. It can be when you're ten pounds or one hundred pounds over where you look and feel good. For me, fat was 5'5" tall and 155 pounds. I looked like somebody had blown me up like a beach ball. I felt awful. It was the summer of '72. I was 21 years old.

Actually, I think I was born at 140 pounds. Not a fat girl, mind you, but big—always too big. People of course said I was just "a big girl," "big-boned," "large-framed." It wasn't true. Underneath it all, once it was truly visible, I was actually rather small-boned with, at most, a medium frame. It had been hidden under all those fat layers.

I never really thought about those fat layers till the summer before college. With the tingling anticipation of new futures and new freedoms came a little voice screaming to have a *little* body. Thus began my dieting "career."

It began with a very sensible, boring diet that lasted all summer. I remember eating cereal and skim milk or two eggs for breakfast, a salad for lunch, and a big steak for dinner.

Well, it worked . . . for a while.

I went down to 116 pounds. I felt skinny. I was ecstatic. *Thin at last!* Unfortunately, it lasted about three months.

After deprivation invariably comes indulgence. I had restricted myself so much that at the first taste of fun, fattening food, I went crazy. I was completely unable to control myself. I shot back up and actually got heavier than I had ever been. I hated it and started trying everything. I did Stillman's diet, Atkins' diet, ice cream diets, banana diets, eat-everything diets, and eat-nothing diets. All of these diets worked; none of them lasted. In my first two years at college, I went from 116 pounds to 155 pounds and back *twice.*

My weight became the theme of my life.

Was I fat? Wasn't I?

Should I eat it? Shouldn't I?

It was a time of *no* cookies or a bagful of cookies and six donuts. I hated it, but I couldn't seem to stop it. On top of it all, I was a nutritional disaster.

Finally, it all crashed to a halt during a routine checkup, by a gynecologist. She was baffled by the different weights she had recorded for me. I explained that they were correct and why. She told me very simply that if I continued on this fat/skinny path, I'd be in the hospital within a year.

I got scared. Everything seemed to depend on being thin: my social life, my self-image, even my career as an actress. But I knew she was right. I was killing myself.

At 155 pounds, my fattest yet, I decided my life was more important than my figure.

I was living at the beach at that time, and amidst the slim bikinied bodies that seemed to be everywhere, I finally decided to accept myself. I decided if I was to be fat, I'd be fat. If a fat lady was to be my role this time around, so be it.

I was sick of it all. I was tired of my own obsession. I wanted to eat whatever I wanted and the hell with it. I was tired of *thinking* about it.

I decided to be healthy and to forget about being thin.

Well, then some very interesting things happened. At first I probably gained a few pounds, but I had ceased to *worry* about it. I no longer weighed myself—in fact, I literally *threw* my scale away. I was fat, but I was free.

I started to look at food in a new way, no longer as the evil tempter but rather as a primary source of nourishment. I got interested in what foods were good for me and why. I bought a wok and slowly started eating a whole new way. I found out I loved lots of vegetables, seafood, and poultry. I started to *feel* better and then gradually, seemingly miraculously, I began to lose weight.

I noticed that I no longer "binged." Instead of a bag of cookies, I could eat a few and forget about them.

Food had stopped being all-important. I ate lots of good, healthy food made mostly in a wok and I enjoyed it. I was no longer deprived, so I no longer had to *stuff*.

By Christmas of that year, I dared to step on a scale. I was down to 132 pounds. Nirvana! I hadn't been trying. I ate whatever I wanted and I was *losing* weight.

I promised myself I wouldn't start thinking about it and jumped off the scale.

By the next summer, I was ready to get on again. I was 125 pounds, a great weight for me.

That was eight years ago. I've never had a weight problem since. I go up and down a few pounds occasionally, but I still have *no* scale. The only time food has gotten out of hand for me in the past few years is when I wanted to be *very* thin, and started to *concentrate* on it too much. When that happens, I catch myself and go back to concentrating on healthy eating and I'm okay again.

When food is in perspective in your head, it will be in proportion on your body. The important thing is to *learn* about food—to learn an easy, simple way to cook and care for yourself that will allow you to be healthy and slim.

Most of us know very little about food. We were taught some vague notions of the four basic food groups and we were raised on white bread, butter, and lots of meat, all tremendously fattening, non-fulfilling foods that many of us continue to eat and then hate ourselves for the inevitable fat they produce. What I have discovered is that once a new consciousness about food is developed, the old fat problems slip away.

So to start, let's forget about the fat/thin aspect of food and concentrate on your . . .

FEELING GOOD!

Together we can let your body be the efficient machine it was created to be. Once you get going on eating well in general, when there's a piece of cake you want, you will be able to eat it and *know* it's okay because nobody ever gained weight from a *treat*. People in America are generally overweight because they live on *over-processed fat foods* that are generally stripped of nutrition. Of *course* they crave and overeat.

Once you get started with brown rice and wokked fresh vegetables, seafood, and poultry, you'll wonder what you ever ate before, and you'll look better than you ever *did* before.

Moreover, you'll *feel* good because your body will be getting what it wants and needs. Pounds will drift away, but let them do *just* that— *drift away*. Think of being slim not *in* two weeks but *for* the rest of your life.

I promise. It worked for me, and I was the worst food fanatic you've ever seen. Now I'm convinced that we weren't *created* to be fat, we were *conditioned* into it.

The emphasis, especially for women, has been placed on skinny bodies instead of glowing faces. Of course we all want to be slim, but we continue to be fat because prolonged deprivation, in an attempt to look like all the magazine pictures crammed down our throats, rarely works.

To start, let yourself be. Forgive yourself. Be proud of yourself *right now*. Know that being fat is not entirely *your* fault and that millions of people share your problem. Know that there *is* a way to be thin without being miserable. If you've tried "everything," why not give yourself one more chance? A very different diet with no calorie count and no scales, a diet not based on punishment but respect and love for oneself. *Food needs to fit into life.* You deserve and need to indulge in and enjoy delicious, satisfying foods. You also owe it to yourself to stop when you have had enough, to think of yourself as special and delicate, to care for yourself with the right foods in the right amounts, to promise yourself not deprivation but an inner awareness of what you really want and need.

I'll never pass up a fresh donut or a home-baked apple pie, but I don't have to anymore. . . .

Once your basic way of eating is healthy and happy, you won't ever again have to pass up anything you *really* want.

FAT HEAD

I've always believed that fat starts in the mind, not in the body. When you're trapped in fat, you don't need another calorie chart or carbohydrate counter. You need a whole new mental picture. So before we actually start using the wok, I thought it important to set some gentle, mental guidelines for your journey into this world of natural, good eating. I've put together the mental guidelines that I feel are responsible for my being a person who is finally thin, who, after years of torment, can put on a pair of size-7 jeans with a sigh of happy disbelief that they fit beautifully. I love being thin, and I'm convinced that anyone can be there, too. No matter what anyone says, it does make an enormous difference in your life. So read the guidelines slowly, then go over them again. They can make the difference in your diet and your state of mind. When you're ready, read on ... having fun learning about woks. New, natural ways of eating can take the emphasis off dieting, and that's very important. Pounds will slip away as you enjoy food more than ever.

A NOTE ABOUT FOOD COMBINING

What you get from food is directly related to what you eat together. Raw foods should be taken at different meals than cooked foods. Liquids should be taken either an hour before or after solid foods, but not together. A protein and a grain are most powerful nutritionally when eaten together. Hot and cold foods should be taken separately. Fruits and vegetables should be taken separately.

THE GENTLE MENTAL GUIDELINES

1. Begin by starting to think of food as a friend, not as an evil tempter. Food is a primary source of nourishment to be carefully selected and slowly savored. A diet that will work forever must be based on respect and love for oneself—not deprivation and punishment.

2. Be aware of everything you put in your mouth. Ask yourself if you really want it, is it good for you, and do you need to eat it now. Remember, you can always have it later or tomorrow or next week. (Food will not have disappeared off the face of the earth by tomorrow!)

3. Eat slowly and delicately and take breaks during your meals to see if you are full. Start to listen to your stomach. It's on your side!

4. If you want a doughnut, eat a *doughnut*. Don't eat out half the refrigerator instead and still want the doughnut. Eat it, enjoy it, and forget about it.

5. Exercise is, of course, important. On days when you are too tired to *do* a lot, be too tired to *eat* a lot.

6. Chew your food extremely well. It makes all the difference. Essential enzymes are released as you masticate your food. Remember, digestion begins in the mouth. Thirty to fifty chews per mouthful is said to be ideal.

7. Forget the idea of three meals a day. Eat when you're hungry, stop when you're full, and don't be afraid to miss a meal occasionally.

8. Never eat if you are angry, excited, upset, in a hurry, or planning to go to bed in the next two hours . . . it's terrible for you!

9. Don't feel you owe anything to anyone when it comes to food. It's your body. If you don't want something, don't eat it. Better to fast than feast in social situations where the food is not right for you.

10. Love yourself a *lot*, no matter what. You are what you've got this time around. Appreciate your progress and forgive your slip-ups. Each day you can begin again. . . .

THE IDEAL DAILY BASIC DIET

If the principle of the four basic food groups never worked for you in practice, take heart. There is a simpler program to base your daily bread on. Dr. Randolph Meltzer, of the Integral Yoga Health Institute in New York City, gave me a program I found easy to remember and foolproof if you follow it.

Each day think of having:

1. One protein
2. One whole grain
3. 65% of your intake vegetables
4. As much raw food as possible

The *protein* may be chosen from cheese, eggs, meat, yogurt, fish, poultry, or beans. For wokking your way skinny, I suggest the less dairy* the better.

The *grain* should be a whole grain and is most important in your diet. Americans are generally lacking in this area. Whole grains supply fiber and work to clean your system.

Vegetables should never get boring. Choose a wide variety and be sure to eat lots of them.

Raw foods contain all the vitamins and minerals they were created with. They also provide roughage to keep the system clear and clean. Think salad at least once a day.

---

* Dairy forms mucus in the body; the less of it you eat, the less phlegm will be in your system. If you feel a cold coming on, stop all dairy and the cold will clear up quickly.

EXERCISE—HOW TO BE A 10!

If you really want to shape up fast, my secret is to always, every possible minute, have an inner awareness of your body. While you sit, stand, walk, or talk, try to be doing something to make your body better. When you bend to pick up something, really use those leg muscles. When you reach for something, stretch out the whole body. The following are a few simpler ideas I use for constant exercise:

On the subway, train, or bus: Forget sitting. Give your seat away and reach for the handstraps. Pull up to your toes and lower yourself down slowly; repeat again and again to get the legs in shape.

While walking: Curve the outside of your feet inward, curl your toes, and really pull yourself along. It's a great leg tightener.

At the beach: Belly lifts while you're sunning! Raise yourself face up on the elbows, lift up the stomach, and, keeping the body straight, lower slowly down.

While carrying something: My friend Arnie Shapiro, who ran the summer house this book was born in, told me the secret for his well-developed chest and arms was also constant exercise awareness, especially when carrying something. A suitcase or a package can give your arms a real workout. Just remember to work both sides of your body equally while you slowly raise and lower the suitcase or package.

In addition to spontaneous exercise, I highly recommend pursuing an interest in a sport or discipline. Yoga, swimming, and rebounding* are my favorites. I find the combination of stretching and tightening is optimum. Running, racquet ball, skating, and karate are all great to keep the muscles moving. Once again, yoga is the perfect accompaniment . . . calming, relaxing, and stretching out the muscles.

---

* Rebounding: A rebounder is a mini trampoline that provides cardiovascular exercise with no chance of injury. I find it to be the perfect urban exercise.

2

WHY A WOK?

A wok fits into this new way of eating because it is the easiest, fastest, most fun way I know of to make delicious meals that will produce a lean, taut body. *It simplifies your kitchen as you simplify your life around eating.* I just can't seem to be thin without one.

Woks lend themselves beautifully to the preparation of naturally slimming foods. Any vegetable can be stir fried in minutes and topped with a little cheese to serve as a delicious, satisfying meal. Fresh seafood can be steamed filleted or whole, poultry can be sliced and stir fried with vegetables to create interesting, delectable meals in minutes. All these dishes are low-calorie, high-energy meals. But when you start to taste how great they are, you won't be eating them because they're low in calories, you'll be eating them because you love how they *taste* and how you *feel* afterward.

And that's how you'll get thin, the *easy* way. When you start feasting on the good stuff, an occasional craving for junk will be fun to satisfy and guilt-free!

Whether you live alone or have a large family, it's easy to wok your way skinny. There's no better way for people, and especially children, to eat.

This style of cooking is as easy for many as it is for one. And the reward for everybody is a happy glow and a healthy, firm body.

Beginner or expert in the kitchen, with this book you can become a Wokmaster practically overnight.

The first step is to realize that a wok is a pot *and* a pan, and that because of its unique shape, it can be used for practically anything. Contrary to many people's preconceptions, it uses little or no *oil*. We'll start out wokking up your morning eggs, wok right through delicious hot lunches and fabulous dinners, and top it all off with light, yummy, *wok-baked* cakes. It's all a part of wokking your way skinny *forever*.

GETTING STARTED—TIPS ON WOK BUYING

Woks are one of the best-selling appliances in this country. This recent surge of wok popularity has brought with it an increased selection to choose from when buying your wok. Woks now come in aluminum, stainless steel, copper, brass, and iron. The best for heating evenly are rolled, tempered steel.

Woks range in size from 12 inches to 26 inches. For everyday home use, 14 to 16 inches is a good-sized selection. It will suit one and serve up to eight. For barbecuing, you might consider a larger size. It's great on the grill.

When shopping for a wok, pick the one that seems most convenient to *you*. Woks are available with one long wooden handle, as well as the traditional wok with two side handles. Some come in sets; if you do not buy a set, be sure to purchase the ring it will rest on over the burner (called the *dok*) and the cover.

And remember, the best place to store your wok is right on top of the stove.

UTENSILS

Your wok may have come with a utensil set. If not, the basics can be purchased separately. For protecting the surface of your wok, I highly recommend the first three below—the other two are just nice to have.

1. The Bamboo Scrubber

   A must for cleaning—easy to use and gentle on the surface

2. Wire Mesh Strainer

   For lifting out foods when deep frying and skimming soups

3. The Flat Lifter

   Great for eggs and omelets—a must for seafood

4. The Ladle

   Like I said, nice to have, but your present ladle will work fine—just never touch the surface of the wok with it

5. Chopsticks

   Great for stirring, but wooden spoons work, too.

WOK ACCESSORIES

1. A chopping board is *absolutely essential,* as well as . . .
2. . . . a good, sharp knife or cleaver, and . . .
3. . . . a small, sharp utility knife.
4. An inexpensive wire whisk will come in really handy at breakfast for whisking eggs.
5. A bamboo or metal steamer.
6. Any kind of little bowls to put sliced vegetables in when setting them aside. It will be easier to add them.

SEASONING YOUR WOK

A most important first step, as seasoning your wok will prevent food from sticking to it. Here is an easy way to season a rolled steel, non-electric wok:

1. Before using, wash it thoroughly. This is the one time Brillo can be used on your wok. Woks are packed in machine oil, which is important to remove.
2. Place wok on its ring (the dok) over burner.

3. Then fill it with hot water and boil for at least two hours over high heat. As it is boiling, continue adding water to the brim—otherwise a watermark will form below the edge.
4. Pour out water. Repeat the process.
5. Dry wok completely over burner over high heat.
6. Next, with several thicknesses of paper toweling moistened with vegetable oil, rub the inside of the wok to close the pores. With fresh towels, repeat until the surface comes away clean. Do this process over medium heat. (Don't panic as you see black on the towels. It's not dirt— just the protective coating the wok is shipped in.)
7. When that's all off, you're ready to begin.
8. If by chance your wok has special or different instructions for seasoning, simply follow them.

To clean wok after each use:

1. Wash with warm sudsy water, then scrub with bamboo brush (available at all housewares stores) or nylon pad.
2. Place wok on dok over burner in upright position.
3. *Dry immediately over high heat.*
4. Let cool down and then rub lightly with 1 teaspoon of oil on a paper towel.

Be faithful in its care and you will be rewarded with a durable, well-seasoned wok.

Woks darken with use—that's part of their charm. They are cherished for their character and memories. You now own an heirloom!

Electric woks need no seasoning because they are precoated with an easy-to-clean, nonstick surface.

3

BECOMING A WOKMASTER

Okay, you've got your wok and it's seasoned. Now it's time to have fun becoming a Wokmaster! The basic concept to understand is that most of the time spent in *Wokcookery* is in the *preparation* of *ingredients*. Everything must be ready *before* you begin heating the wok, for once you begin the cooking time is a matter of moments. So slice everything you will be using and put it into individual little bowls. Have your oil and seasonings out and ready. Then it's as easy as one, two, three.

THE BASIC PRINCIPLE

One: Heat the wok over high heat.

Two: Once it is hot (2 to 3 minutes), make a necklace of oil around the top of the wok. It will slide down, coating the sides and leaving a little pool in the bottom.

Three: Immediately start adding ingredients and stir.

Congratulations—you've begun!

ON HEAT

Wokcookery can be done over gas or electric heat. However, if you are using an electric stove, you must be especially careful about temperature control. Instead of preheating your wok over high heat, use medium-high, since it will be impossible to quickly bring the heat down. The wok is designed for both gas and electric stoves. For gas stoves, place larger-diameter circle down; simply flip over for electric stoves.

ON DIAGONAL SLICING

Diagonal slicing is an Oriental tradition, and with good reason. By slicing with your knife at a 45-degree angle to the food, you produce thin slices that expose the largest possible area to heat, contributing to a fast cooking time. It is ideal in Wokcookery, since the cooking is done over high heat. Use this method for meats and fibrous vegetables and it will also help tenderize them.

BASIC METHODS OF WOKCOOKERY

1. *Stir frying* is exactly that. It's simply heating the wok, necklacing with oil, and tossing in the vegetables. Stir to coat with oil and keep stirring until vegetables are firm but tender. This method prevents loss of vitamins in water and never lets veggies get limp. The color of the vegetables will actually deepen and brighten beautifully.

People often ask me if stir frying isn't fattening because of "all the oil you use." I'd like to clear that up right now. When you stir fry, you are merely *necklacing* the sides of the wok with a *drizzle* of oil. When the seasoning (the patina) on your wok has built up, you can actually stir fry without *any* oil. However, it's important to know that the use of small amounts of oil is incredibly valuable in your diet. Oil *lubricates* your entire system. One to two tablespoons a day is essential to keep your body flowing smoothly.

Now because that oil is so valuable, the *kind* of oil you use is also very important. A good oil is a pure (if possible, cold-pressed) oil without a lot of preservatives. Corn, peanut, safflower, sunflower, and sesame are all good for you and are very high in protein. Cheap, over-processed vegetable oils are usually a collection of odds and ends in which nothing is left of value to you.

2. *Steaming.* For three dollars you can turn your wok into a hassle-free steamer. A stainless steel insert can be purchased and fit right into your wok when you want to steam. You just boil water in the wok, put in the insert, and lay your vegetables, fish, or whatever on top, and cover. I discovered a round cake rack also works fine, and you probably have one already. You can also buy tiered wooden steamers, which work well and can steam several dishes at once. Your wok may have come with two wooden crisscrossed sticks for steaming. They fit in the bottom, and, again, you boil water beneath them in the wok and lay vegetables across in a heat-proof server. They work okay, but the three-dollar stainless steel type can't be beat. Steaming adds no calories and also loses no vitamins.

3. *Poaching.* Poaching fish is an easy, fine-tasting method of preparation. It is especially good for whole fish, but large thick fillets wrapped in a porous cloth will work well also. The wok's shape makes it ideal for poaching since the thickest part (the center) of the fish will be closest to the flame, allowing the whole fish to be cooked perfectly in the same amount of time.

To Poach Fish: In your wok, bring to boil enough water to totally cover fish by 1 inch. Then lower the heat so that the water is just below the boiling point, and place the fish in the wok. Cover and adjust the heat to lowest possible setting. Cook 10 minutes for a 12-inch fish, and lift out.

Again, poaching is a low-calorie, highly nutritional kind of preparation. On page 116 you'll discover the joys of Poached Salmon with Yogurt Dill Sauce.

4. *Tempura/Deep Frying.* Tempura is a Japanese method of preparation in which pieces of vegetables and fish are coated with a light,

chilled batter and dropped into very hot oil. It is similar to, but not exactly, what Americans have come to know as deep frying. The difference is that with tempura the batter-covered vegetables and fish are so cold and the oil in the wok so hot that there is no chance of the oil being heavily absorbed. The intense and well-distributed heat immediately seals the nutrients and flavors into the food, assuring a light, especially nongreasy result.

Now tempura is a treat. It is heavier than most anything else made in the wok. I wouldn't suggest eating it every night, but as a specialty for once in a while it's fun to make and great to taste. I've created an especially light tempura batter for you as you wok your way skinny. The recipe for it starts on page 111.

5. *Soup Making.* Because of its size and well-distributed heat, your wok is great for soups. However, if you are going to do a lot of soup making in the wok, I recommend your purchasing a second wok, for the long simmering process can eventually break down the patina (seasoned surface). With two woks, you can keep one for soup making, poaching, steaming, and cake baking, and reserve the other for stir frying and egg dishes.

A big jar of wokked soup is a great thing to have around, especially in winter. It will fill you up and not out. Recipes in the soup section will show you have to turn leftover veggies into elegant crocks of steaming soup.

6. *Barbecuing.* Bring your wok outside and on the road! It works great over a barbecue grill or hibachi. When camping, simply dig a fire pit and straddle the dok across it. Place the wok on the dok and you're all set.

Now you don't have to be stuck with boring, fattening food like hot dogs and hamburgers. You can even wok your way skinny traveling across the country!

7. *Cake Baking.* That's right, you can actually "bake" cakes in it— *steam* bake, that is. As the pounds drift away and you're looking for a yummy light dessert, you can turn to page 137, where a whole section on sweetness awaits. Each of the dessert recipes that I've created in this book is designed for the Wokmaster on a new, skinny path. All of them are light and low in fat, but you'd never know it by how good they taste!

4

RECIPES

In my first book of Wokcookery, there are many dishes that are light to eat and easy to make. Once you are steadily losing or at the right weight for you, you can delve into it for lots more exciting ideas in Wokcookery. This book, however, was created specifically for the *losing* of weight while you get healthy. All of these recipes were created for *wokkin' your way skinny.*

Enjoy!

HOW TO READ A RECIPE

In these carefully tested, original recipes, you will find all the ingredients listed first, followed by the preparation, which is written simply step by step. So just . . .

1. Read through the recipe to get a general idea of the preparation.
2. Check to make sure you have all the ingredients.

3. Put out all the ingredients and have them ready as specified.
4. Follow the numerically listed steps.
5. Enjoy the tasty rewards.

A beginner in the kitchen or an expert can meet with fun and success. If you've got any ideas about being a lousy cook, just forget them! Anyone can do it, and you're already on your way.

YIELD

When you decide to make a recipe, one of the first things to figure out is how many people you are preparing for and how much the recipe yields as listed. It sounds simple enough, but if you've ever made a recipe that the author felt fed four and in reality fed only two of *your* hungry guests, you have an idea of what I'm talking about.

Everybody eats differently and has different notions of what it means to feed a family. In some families, one serving is all anyone ever wants; in others, two or three servings are commonplace. Now I happen to like food to be plentiful. You will find that wokked food is light, so you can eat more and it all keeps beautifully in the refrigerator for tasty leftovers. Therefore, I have chosen to write these recipes for *hungry* people and on each recipe a yield is given. All of them can be easily adapted to your particular needs.

Remember, it's better to eat as much as you need of the wokked delight so that you will not be tempted to eat a loaf of bread along with it.

A WORD ABOUT PROTEIN

When people talk about "*needing* a lot of red meat," I know the feeling they are talking about. It's a craving for protein. But red meat is not the only and far from the best way of filling that craving.

Consider some facts about the glorified steak:

First, it is the only thing that takes longer than 24 hours to digest. That means that the "beautiful steak" you eat at dinner is desperately trying to be digested by your body all that night and all the next day. That's a long time for so much energy to be funneled to your stomach. It can make you feel sluggish.

Second, it's high, very high, in calories. On top of which, nutritionists are starting to discover just how bad a lot of meat is for you.

Now that doesn't mean you should *never* eat meat. If you love it and want it, eat it—but *once in a while,* or eat it "wok style," which means sliced in slender strips and stir fried with lots of veggies.

Luckily, fine alternatives do exist to fill that craving for protein. Fresh seafood and poultry are very high in protein, low in calories, and easy on your system. If you are now a big meat eater, try substituting a lot of seafood and poultry and see if you don't feel a difference. Once you discover that light feeling, even right after eating, red meat will be a lot easier to pass up.

Another excellent source of protein is brown rice. To start off, it's a perfect complement to wok dinners. It's also a good protein source, especially as a partner to beans, tofu, or nuts.

On top of which, it's so very cheap!

The best kind to buy is short-grain brown rice, which is sold in bulk at all natural food stores. If that is unavailable to you, you can buy boxed brown rice in most supermarkets.

Brown rice is not at all the same as white rice. There is nothing left in white rice—they took the good stuff all out to make it pretty.

How much brown rice you start eating depends a lot on you, but some brown rice in your diet is practically essential. It is a whole grain. It is both the seed and the fruit of the grass plant. Within it are all the essential elements for a new life cycle. It contains not only protein but calcium, iron, phosphorus, thiamine, riboflavin, and niacin. It's low in cholesterol, contains only a trace of fat, and is veritably free of saturated fats. It is also especially easy to digest because of its low fiber content.

All this for 55 cents a pound!!!

By keeping a nice big bowl of brown rice in your refrigerator, you will have the basis for any meal. It's great stir fried next to eggs when you crave hash browns, stir fried with vegetables for quick fried rice, or warmed up to go under any wokked delight.

The following is my favorite, failproof recipe for brown rice sold in bulk:

ANNIE'S RICE

Put on 4 cups of water* to boil in your teakettle. Meanwhile, rinse 2⅓ cups of short-grain brown rice in cold water. In a heavy saucepan, heat 1 tablespoon of oil. Add rice and saute over low heat until the moisture is absorbed and rice smells nutty.

Add the 4 cups boiling water and 1 teaspoon salt to rice (1 tablespoon soy sauce or tamari may also be added). Allow to boil uncovered for 2 to 3 minutes. DO NOT STIR. Then cover, reduce heat to very low, and allow to cook for 45 minutes. Do *not* open or stir. After 45 minutes turn off heat, but let rice sit unopened for 15 more minutes.

Then fluff gently with fork and serve.

It is important not to stir the rice because rice stacks up one grain on top of the other. By stirring, you break the casings that surround the grain and the rice becomes sticky.

Store in your refrigerator loosely covered.

Be sure to really *chew* brown rice, since a lot of its sweetness is then released and it also aids the digestive process.

SEEDS

Seeds—sesame, poppy, and caraway—are also a protein source and add a good, nutty flavor to dishes. Unhulled sesame seeds are the best. Toast in a dry frying pan or wok until they start to pop; cool and store in a jar. They are a great natural seasoning and are available in natural food stores.

* Water can be replaced with soup stock for extra flavor and nourishment.

TAMARI

Tamari is a natural version of soy sauce and I think it tastes even better. It is available in natural food stores and can be used interchange-
ably with soy sauce in any recipe.

TAHINI

Tahini is a paste made from ground sesame seeds. It is available in natural food stores and well worth trying.

5

Good Morning!

TIME FOR BREAKFAST IN YOUR WOK!

Now it's time to really get cooking, and I think breakfast is the best place to start. If you *never* eat breakfast, try out these recipes for brunch. All that talk about breakfast being important is very true. You haven't eaten in at least 8 hours, and if you want to get going, you've got to put something in your stomach that will boost you.

All these recipes will put a zip in your day and also will keep you full for hours. If you must have bread with your eggs, forget white bread. A slice of whole wheat or protein bread is at least more than just empty starch.

See if you really need that second piece of bread—or if it's just a habit. Bread is bulk; if you're really hungry, try a little brown rice stir fried on the side.

If you have no time or appetite in the morning, reach for fresh fruit either by itself or with cottage cheese or yogurt. Forget danishes, coffee, and buttered bagels! (If you gave your dog a danish, coffee, and a cigarette every morning, would you really expect him to live??)

And if we're talking about breakfast, I can't resist . . .

A NOTE ABOUT EGGS

Remember how different eggs used to look? Big bright yellow yolks and thick whites? They tasted better then, too.

Years ago all chickens produced fertile, natural eggs. That means the hens were really impregnated by roosters. It was also a time when hens and roosters ate real grain and were allowed to run free in the sun.

Well, unfortunately, the eggs you buy in the supermarket today no longer come from such happy homes. To speed up everything and make more money, hens are now artificially inseminated, fed chemicals, and made to reside indoors under bright lights that create 12-hour days.

More eggs quicker means more money for the egg sellers.

Unfortunately, it also means less of everything for you and me—and nobody even told us! Less taste and less nutrition are passed on to us as well as a lot more chemicals.

Real eggs can be found in your natural food store. There are thousands of them across the country—check out your area. Their eggs are marked NATURAL, FERTILE eggs. When cracked open, they look and taste the way eggs *used* to . . . bright yellow yolks, thick whites, great flavor.

SCALLIONED SESAME EGGS

INGREDIENTS:

4 eggs
1 tablespoon milk or water
1 teaspoon sesame seeds
1 scallion (also called spring onion!)
    salt and pepper to taste
    oil for cooking (sesame is especially good if you have it)

1. Rinse and chop scallion. Set aside.
2. Beat eggs with milk or water and salt and pepper.
3. Heat wok.
4. Necklace with oil.
5. Add scallion and sesame seeds and stir fry for 2 to 3 minutes.
6. Add eggs and continue stirring until they are desired consistency.
7. Lift out and enjoy.

SERVES 2

39

FRESH STRAWBERRY MUENSTER CHEESE OMELET

INGREDIENTS:

4–6 whole fresh strawberries
4 eggs
1 tablespoon milk or water
  salt and pepper to taste
2 very thin slices muenster cheese
  oil for cooking

1. Rinse and quarter strawberries. Set aside.
2. Beat eggs with milk or water and salt and pepper.
3. Heat wok.
4. Necklace with oil.
5. Stir fry strawberries for 1 minute.
6. Add eggs and continue stirring to almost desired consistency.
7. Flip eggs and lay cheese across eggs.
8. Sprinkle sides of wok with cold water to create steam. Cover immediately.
9. When cheese is melted, lift out.
10. Serve.

SERVES 2

ZUCCHINI AND EGGS

INGREDIENTS:

1 scallion
1 small–medium zucchini
3 eggs
1 tablespoon milk or water
1 teaspoon sesame seeds
  salt and pepper to taste
  oil for cooking
  optional: a sprinkle of fresh basil and/or a topping of 2 tablespoons grated cheddar cheese

1. Rinse and chop scallion. Set aside.
2. Wash zucchini carefully (they're sandy) and slice in thin circles. Set aside.
3. Beat eggs with milk or water and salt and pepper.
4. Heat wok.
5. Necklace with oil.
6. Stir fry scallion for 1 minute.
7. Add zucchini and sesame seeds, sprinkle with salt and pepper (and add basil, if using).
8. Stir fry zucchini until golden.
9. Add eggs. Stir fry all together. (Add cheese, if using,) and steam melt.
10. Cook till desired consistency. Lift out and serve.

SERVES 2

SUPER STEVEN'S SURPRISE

Without my friend Steven Joseph, not only this omelet but this book might never have seen the light of day. His unflagging support of this project and this author caused this book to be born in a beautiful seaside resort called Kismet on New York's Fire Island. Because of him, instead of creating and testing (i.e., sweating!) alone over a hot stove in Manhattan all summer I was able to share the beach and these creations with a summer family of friends—many of whom turned out to be Wokmasters in their own right. Steven is one of them. Steven never thought he could cook and then gradually began to play in the kitchen. Realizing how easy and how much fun it is, he went on to become my #1 collaborator in our daily meals, which fed from four to fourteen people! Steven's greatest asset lies in his knack for improvisation: on a day when even I thought there was nothing in the refrigerator, he whipped up an omelet that surprised us all. Have fun trying this for your own breakfast surprise!

INGREDIENTS:

 2 carrots, grated
 1 onion, finely sliced
 1 tablespoon sesame seeds
 1 handful alfalfa sprouts
 4 eggs, beaten
   salt and pepper to taste
   oil for cooking

1. Heat wok.
2. Necklace with oil.
3. Stir fry carrots and onion till tender.
4. Add alfalfa sprouts and sesame seeds and stir fry.
5. Add eggs. Season with salt and pepper.
6. Keep moving eggs around wok.
7. Cook till desired consistency and serve.

SERVES 2

THE TIMBALE STORY

By definition the word *timbale* comes from the Arab *thabal,* meaning "drum," a small metal receptacle that is round in shape and is intended to hold a beverage.

These days the term has been stretched to include dishes cooked and served in a pie crust as well as foods prepared and served in small cups or containers. Our Timbales are crust-free and steamed in the wok. We find them to be an interesting change of pace. They have the feel of something decadent, but they're actually light, very healthy, and perfect for wokking your way skinny!

COTTAGE CHEESE TIMBALES

INGREDIENTS:

    2 large eggs, beaten in 2-cup measuring cup
4–5 ounces milk
    pinch of salt
    pinch of pepper
    pinch of nutmeg
    2 ounces (½ cup) cottage cheese
    1 tablespoon tahini (sesame paste)
    2 tablespoons minced scallion (or snipped fresh chives)
    1 teaspoon butter

1. Beat eggs in measuring cup until well blended.
2. Add 4 to 5 ounces milk or enough to make 1 cup of egg-milk mixture.
3. Add salt, pepper, nutmeg, cottage cheese, tahini, and scallion or chives.
4. Blend well.
5. Pour mixture into 2 buttered ramekins, custard cups, or other suitable containers.
6. Dot top of each with ½ teaspoon butter.
7. Place on steamer rack set over simmering water in wok. Cover and steam 20 to 25 minutes until mixture is firm and knife inserted in center comes out clean.

SERVES 2

SKIP'S BLOODY MARY EGGS

I met Skip Skwarek in the final months of compiling my first book. He came in, rolled up his sleeves, and helped me perfect and test the final recipes. He also contributed some of his own wonderful creations to the list. Next you'll find his Bloody Mary Eggs—and are they great!

INGREDIENTS:

- 2 large eggs
- 5 ounces tomato puree (or juice—but puree is better)
- ½ cup minced celery (use leaves, too)
- 2 teaspoons Worcestershire sauce
- ¼ teaspoon Tabasco, or to taste
- 1 tablespoon fresh snipped dill (or 1 teaspoon dried)
- 1 teaspoon butter

1. Beat eggs until frothy, then beat in tomato puree or juice.
2. Add celery, Worcestershire, Tabasco, and dill. Blend well.
3. Pour into 2 buttered ramekins, custard cups, or other suitable containers.
4. Dot each with ½ teaspoon butter.
5. Place on steamer rack set over simmering water in wok. Cover and steam 20 to 25 minutes until mixture is firm and knife inserted in center comes out clean.

SERVES 2

THE STORY OF TOFU

Have you ever been at an Oriental vegetable stand and noticed little white cakes floating in water? Ever wonder what they were? Well, they're tofu! And now tofu is available in most supermarkets.

Tofu is a fermented bean curd made from soybeans, and as strange as it sounds, tofu is really something very special. The texture is that of soft cheese and the flavor is fairly bland, but tofu's great asset is that it quickly absorbs the flavor of whatever it is in. Best of all, it is very high in protein and very low in calories! It also costs literally pennies to serve. I call it "future steak" and predict that ten years from now almost everyone will know and appreciate tofu. It is really something to get hooked on. It is available in both large and small curd. The large squares are Japanese; the smaller, Chinese. Both have the same flavor, but the texture is a little different. I suggest you try them both. When I make spaghetti sauce, I always blend in chunks of tofu with the sauce to fortify a pasta dish with protein. It's also delicious blended as a salad dressing or vegetable dip.

The wonders of tofu are woven throughout this book. On the next page you'll find Tofu Scrambled Eggs, a mock scrambled egg dish that's delicious.

Note: Tofu should be stored in a container covered with fresh, cool water. Change the water every day. Storage time is one week for optimum flavor. It can also be frozen. To remove excess moisture from tofu cakes, place each cake on the underside of a flat-bottomed plate. Top with another flat-bottomed plate. Hold over sink at an angle and press plates firmly together until moisture stops dripping out.

To achieve a chewier texture with tofu, squeeze out moisture as described above. Wrap tofu so that it is airtight and freeze for 48 to 72 hours. When ready to use, thaw tofu in refrigerator for 6 to 8 hours or in a bowl of lukewarm water for 1 hour.

TOFU SCRAMBLED EGGS

INGREDIENTS:

4 Chinese or
2 Japanese bean curd cakes (tofu), mashed with fork
2 scallions, finely chopped
1 tablespoon sesame seeds
1 tablespoon tamari, or soy sauce
  pinch of saffron (for egg yellow color!)
  oil for cooking

1. Heat wok.
2. Necklace with oil.
3. Add scallions and sesame seeds. Stir fry for 1 minute.
4. Add tofu and mix together.
5. Season with tamari and saffron.
6. Serve.

SERVES 2

A SHOUT ABOUT SPROUTS!

What's packed with vitamin C, practically calorie-free, and able to grow in your kitchen cupboard? Sprouts—an amazing thing to know about, a virtual dieter's delight. Sprouts are the offshoots of seeds and beans, and almost any of them can be sprouted. Super-energy food, sprouts can be added to almost any wokked dish, served as lettuce on a sandwich, or made into a lovely salad—and you can have a constant supply on your kitchen shelf! I've included simple instructions for growing your own—it's fun and easy. Alfalfa and mung bean sprouts also can be purchased packaged in natural food stores.

SPROUT IT YOURSELF

THE JAR METHOD:

You will need:

1 quart glass jar
1 piece of cheesecloth or nylon netting
1 rubber band or canning jar ring
    seeds (about ¼ cup)
    water

1. Put seeds in quart jar, cover with warm water, and soak overnight.
2. In the morning, place a piece of cheesecloth or nylon netting over the top of the jar, secure it with a rubber band or canning jar ring, and drain off excess water.
3. Put the jar on its side and place in a warm, dark place (like your cupboard).
4. Two or three times a day, rinse the seeds with water and drain well. Put the jar back on its side in the cupboard.
5. Your crop will be ready in 3 or 4 days. Then place the jar on the windowsill and let the sprouts have light for one day so they can begin making chlorophyll.
6. Eat and enjoy! Refrigerate those sprouts you're not going to eat at once and don't forget to begin the next crop!

SPROUTS ARE READY TO EAT WHEN THEY REACH THESE SIZES:

Alfalfa	1 inch
Chick peas	½ to ¾ inch
Flaxseed	¾ inch
Lentil	1 inch
Mung	1½ to 2½ inches
Soybean	½ inch

THE SHOUT SPROUT OMELET

INGREDIENTS:

2 handfuls of your favorite homegrown sprouts
8 cherry tomatoes
4 eggs, beaten
　pinch of fresh or dried basil
½ cup grated cheddar cheese
　oil for cooking
　salt and pepper to taste

1. Heat wok.
2. Necklace with oil.
3. Stir fry sprouts for 1 minute.
4. Add tomatoes and basil. Stir fry gently.
5. Add eggs, and salt and pepper to taste.
6. Stir fry till eggs are almost desired consistency.
7. Sprinkle with cheese.
8. Sprinkle sides of wok with cold water, then cover and steam to melt cheese.
9. Serve.

SERVES 2

ANNIE'S ROLLED OATS

Something happens when you eat Annie's Rolled Oats in the morning. You sort of glow all day—your stomach feels so good, so calm, so satisfied. I couldn't make it through the winter without Annie's Rolled Oats!

INGREDIENTS:

   1 cup oats
   1 tablespoon oil for cooking
2¼ cups boiling water
     dash of tamari or soy sauce
 ¼ cup bran
     dash of cinnamon
 ¼ cup raisins
 ½ teaspoon vanilla

1. Toast oats in oil till they smell sweet and toasty (but are not brown).
2. Turn off oats and oil, then add 2¼ cups boiling water to wok.
3. Turn heat back on under wok. Bring oats and water to boil, add bran, raisins, cinnamon, and vanilla slowly, and stir and cover.
4. Simmer 15 minutes over low heat.
5. Add dash of tamari. Stir in.
6. Cook 5 minutes more and serve.

For variation: Replace ¼ cup of bran with bulgur and toast with oats for denser oatmeal texture.

SERVES 2

JOEL'S BREAKFAST DELIGHT

A musician who became in tune with his body, Joel created a breakfast delight that sticks to your ribs and is packed with vitamins and protein. On a cold winter's morning, it's a sure hit!

INGREDIENTS:

oil for cooking
1 cup 7-grain cereal (available packaged in natural food stores)
½ cake bean curd, cut into small pieces
1 tablespoon wheat germ
1 tablespoon coconut
1 teaspoon cinnamon
2 tablespoons raisins
1 tablespoon sesame seeds
2 cups boiling water
1 banana

1. Heat wok over low heat.
2. Necklace with oil.
3. Toast cereal with sesame seeds and wheat germ till golden.
4. Add boiling water and rest of ingredients except banana.
5. Cover and lower heat. Simmer 15 minutes, stirring occasionally.
6. Add banana and cook 5 minutes more. Serve.

SERVES 2

52

6

LUNCH AT HOME

If you're a big breakfast eater, lunch can be as simple as a cup of soup from the deli or a fresh salad.

However, if you're one of the many who can't face food in the morning or don't have the time to cook breakfast, lunch becomes the first real meal of the day. On the next pages you'll find hot lunches to eat at home and yummy cold dishes to pack up and bring to work.

When you do order out or go out to lunch, try to stay away from sandwiches—all that bread is heavy on the stomach, especially if you'll be sitting a lot after lunch. I very often order breakfast when everyone else is getting lunch.

Again, eat as much as *feels* right. Light lunches will make for energetic days.

FRESH ASPARAGUS WITH DILL AND BABY JARLSBERG

If you're lucky enough to be home for a hot lunch, this is a perfect midday meal. It's also a great dinner with hot brown rice on the side.

INGREDIENTS:

        1 bunch fresh asparagus
    1–2 tablespoons fresh dill
        ½ cup grated baby Jarlsberg cheese
            salt and pepper to taste
            oil for cooking

1. Wash asparagus and remove bottom 1 inch of stalks. Diagonal-slice the entire rest of stalks into fairly thin pieces, leaving the top 2 inches whole. Set aside.
2. Finely chop dill. Set aside.
3. Grate cheese. Set aside.
4. Heat wok.
5. Necklace with oil.
6. Add asparagus and dill. Season with salt and pepper. Stir fry 3 to 5 minutes till crisp-tender.
7. Sprinkle with cheese.
8. Sprinkle sides of wok with cold water to create steam.
9. Cover. When cheese is melted, it's ready!

SERVES 2

SPAGHETTI SQUASH

When you live at the beach, a recurring theme, especially with the ladies, is pounds versus pasta. (Is it ever really worth it?) Well, once our summer house discovered spaghetti squash, we had the problem licked. It is a large yellow squash which contains a pulp of long spaghetti-like strings. Spaghetti squash tastes much like pasta—only it's not fattening at all! We think "pretend pasta" is the best, and it's as easy as 1, 2, 3!

INGREDIENTS:

1 large spaghetti squash
1 quart tomato sauce, heated
  Parmesan cheese

1. Place steamer rack in wok and pour boiling water beneath rack.
2. Split open squash and place both halves on rack. Cover wok and steam squash till tender (45 minutes to 1 hour).
3. When "spaghetti" pulls out of squash skin easily, it's ready. Pull out with fork, place in bowl, top with tomato sauce, and serve with Parmesan cheese.

SERVES 2–4

TOFU TACOS FOR TWO

That's right—vegetarian tacos! Decadent and delicious!

INGREDIENTS:

            2 cakes tofu (Chinese or small curd is best)
    ⅛–¼ teaspoon saffron, salt, basil, thyme
        ⅛ teaspoon curry, or to taste
        1 clove pressed garlic
        1 teaspoon sesame seeds
        1 tablespoon tamari or soy sauce, to taste
        ¼ cup Parmesan cheese
        1 tomato
        1 cup shredded lettuce
        2 chopped scallions (optional)
            taco shells or pita pockets
            oil for cooking

1. Cut tofu into ½-inch slices and pat out excess water with absorbent towel. Then cut into cubes.
2. Heat wok over high heat.
3. Necklace with oil.
4. Add tofu and stir fry for 3 minutes. Lower to medium heat.
5. Add saffron and stir fry till tofu is yellow.
6. Add rest of seasonings, sesame seeds, and garlic. Stir fry.
7. Add oil if necessary to prevent sticking.
8. Put heat back up. Add 1 tablespoon tamari, or to taste.
9. Stir constantly and add cheese. When cheese melts, serve in tacos or pita pockets topped with lettuce, tomato, and scallions.

SERVES 2

MEET ME AT SOUEN

Of all the places in the world one might live, residing next to a restaurant such as Souen is a most fortunate thing. Souen is considered to be one of the finest macrobiotic restaurants not only in New York City but in the world. It opened twelve years ago on New York's Upper West Side (on Broadway between 89th and 90th streets), and for a long time I didn't know it was there. I stumbled in one day and I've been addicted ever since.

First of all, everything in there is great for you—not just good but great: the freshest of vegetables, the most delicate of fish, savory sauces, thick homemade soups, and outrageous sugar-free desserts. No preservatives, sugar, or dairy are used, the principle of the food preparation being based on macrobiotics—*macro* meaning "large," *biotic* meaning "life." Souen's very reasonable prices make it easy to rationalize eating out a lot. The practically calorie-free Yudofu is the next recipe.

A restaurant such as this is a service to the neighborhood it is so much a part of. When I'm in New York, my first stop is Souen. There are now two Souens. The second, recent addition is downtown (on Broadway and Prince Street). It is a culinary experience not to be missed. Thank you, Yama. Thank you, Kate. And a big thank you to the entire Souen staff. You're terrific!

SOUEN'S YUDOFU

INGREDIENTS:

    1 cup shredded carrots
    1 cup shredded cabbage
      handful watercress
    1 cup broccoli
    2 large cakes of tofu (Japanese is great here)

DIPPING SAUCE:

    1 tablespoon fresh minced ginger
    1 finely chopped scallion
    ½ cup tamari or soy sauce
    ½ cup water for broth

1. Arrange vegetables and tofu in casserole. Start with carrots and cabbage on bottom, add broccoli and watercress, top with tofu in middle. Then slice tofu.
2. Fill casserole halfway with water and place on steamer rack in wok.
3. Place boiling water under rack and boil covered till veggies are bright and crisp-tender.
4. Combine all sauce ingredients and serve together.

SERVES 2

CAPONATA

Caponata could be considered a Sicilian-Italian Ratatouille, just slightly tarter. It can be served hot or cold, as an appetizer or main dish. It even works well as a stuffing for eggplant, peppers, or squash. It can be served over rice or pasta and can also be used in combination with chicken for a zesty dish. You'll find a Chicken Caponata, inspired by my Sicilian Grandmother Antoinette Viscardi, on page 100.

INGREDIENTS:

         oil for cooking
    1 pound eggplant, unpeeled, diced in 1-inch cubes
    1 cup onion, thinly sliced
    1 cup celery, thinly sliced
    ½ cup Italian sweet green pepper, cored, seeded, and coarsely chopped
    2 cups tomatoes, chopped (and peeled for truly elegant results)
    4 tablespoons capers, drained and coarsely chopped
    4 tablespoons pignoli nuts, finely chopped
10–12 Italian or Greek black olives (cured in brine), pitted and coarsely chopped
    1 teaspoon oregano
    ¼ teaspoon crushed dried red pepper
    ¼ cup fresh basil, chopped (or 2 teaspoons dried)
    ¼ cup parsley, chopped
    ¼ cup red wine or cider vinegar
    2 tablespoons honey (optional)
       lemon wedges

1. Heat wok over high heat and necklace with oil.
2. Stir fry eggplant in several batches until somewhat browned and softened. Remove to a bowl and reserve.
3. Add a bit more oil to wok. Add onion, celery, and green pepper and stir fry several minutes until onions are translucent.
4. Add tomatoes, capers, nuts, olives, oregano, crushed red pepper, and basil. Simmer uncovered for 5 to 7 minutes to blend flavors.
5. Add reserved eggplant, cover, and simmer for 5 minutes or until eggplant is *al dente*.
6. Add parsley, vinegar, and optional honey. Simmer uncovered for several minutes.
7. Serve hot or cold, garnished with lemon wedges.

SERVES 4

A NEW KIND OF BURGER

How about Kasha Burgers for lunch? Or Tofu Burgers on the barbecue grill? Lower in fat and calories than meat, these vegetarian burgers are crowd pleasers. If you make them in large quantities over the weekend, you can use the leftovers for lunch during the week and freeze them—replacing the traditional (fattening) hamburger with a truly unique delight.

TOFU BURGERS

INGREDIENTS:

1 large cake tofu (or 2 Chinese small curd cakes), drained and crumbled
½ cup bran
¼ cup toasted wheat germ
2 tablespoons tamari or soy sauce
¼ teaspoon chili powder, or to taste
½ cup shredded carrots
1 scallion, finely minced
  optional: serve with 4 small size pita pockets or 2 large pockets cut in half, 4 tomato slices, and 1 cup sprouts

1. Press excess water from tofu.
2. Place tofu in bowl and crumble with fork.
3. Add bran, wheat germ, tamari, chili powder, carrots, and scallion. Mix well and form into 4 patties.
4. Heat wok.
5. Necklace with oil.
6. When oil is hot, place patties in two at a time.
7. Flip when golden (about 2 to 3 minutes).
8. Remove patties and place on platter in warm oven. Repeat till all patties are done.
9. Serve inside pita pockets topped with sprouts, tomato slices, and perhaps a tablespoon of your favorite salad dressing or condiment.

MAKES 4 TOFUBURGERS

JOHN AND ANNIE'S KASHA BURGERS

Annie Fox and John Clark should probably win an award for "new age couple of the year." Based in New York, their combined effort in the whole-food field is bringing new and important information to us all. If something ails you, chances are John and Annie can fix it. They are at least ten years ahead of their time.

Their influence expanded my direction and understanding of diet and nutrition immeasurably. Someday their work will be available to you directly. Till then I'm honored to have several of their recipes be part of this book. (Annie Fox/John Clark Whole Foods, 45 East 45th Street, Suite 709, New York, N.Y. 212 730-7026)

INGREDIENTS:

    1 large cake tofu, pressed
    ¾ cup kasha
    2 tablespoons tamari or soy sauce
    ¼ cup celery, finely chopped
    ¼ cup onion, finely chopped
    2 cloves garlic, minced
    ¼ teaspoon Italian herbs, thyme, basil, oregano
      dash of sage
      oil for cooking
      optional: serve with pita pockets, tomato slices, sprouts, and condiments

1. Heat wok.
2. Necklace with oil.
3. Stir fry celery, onion, and garlic till tender. Let cool.
4. Crumble tofu in bowl with fork.
5. Add to bowl kasha, tamari, cooked veggies, and seasoning. Mix well.
6. Form into 4 patties.
7. Heat wok again.
8. Necklace with oil.
9. Cook patties two at a time. Serve on lettuce or stuff in pita pockets and top with sprouts, tomatoes, and favorite condiments.

Note: All burgers are also great broiled.

MAKES **4** LARGE PATTIES

MY MAMA'S TUNA ZUCCHINI BURGERS ON A BED OF LETTUCE

INGREDIENTS:

oil for cooking
¼ pound zucchini, coarsely grated (about 1 cup firmly packed)
1 small onion, grated or finely minced
⅓ cup bulgur
2 ounces mushrooms, finely minced (about ½ cup)
¼ cup lemon juice (juice from 1 lemon)
3 tablespoons tamari or soy sauce
¼ teaspoon hot chili oil, Tabasco, or cayenne pepper
¼ cup fresh snipped dill (or 2 teaspoons dried)
1 6½-ounce can tuna in water, drained and flaked
1 large egg, lightly beaten
¾ pound mung bean sprouts, well drained
lettuce leaves for garnish

1. In a bowl, combine well the zucchini, onion, bulgur, mushrooms, lemon juice, 1 tablespoon tamari, chili oil, dill, and tuna. Let marinate for 20 minutes to 1 hour until bulgur has absorbed liquid and softened.
2. Mix in beaten egg.
3. Form into 6 small patties, the thinner the better.
4. Heat wok over high heat and necklace with oil.
5. Fry patties, three at a time, for 2 to 3 minutes on each side until nicely browned and crusty. Remove from wok and keep warm.
6. Add sprouts and 2 tablespoons tamari to wok and stir fry 1 minute until heated through.
7. To serve, place a large lettuce leaf on each plate. Put some sprouts on each leaf and top sprouts with 2 tuna patties per serving.

MAKES 6 SMALL PATTIES

PINACH SUPREME

INGREDIENTS:

6 large mushrooms
3 asparagus spears, if available
1 clove garlic, minced, or ¼ teaspoon garlic powder
2 squares tofu
   pinch basil
2 tablespoons sesame seeds, toasted
   tamari or soy sauce to taste
5 teaspoons fresh ground pepper
   oil for cooking
1 bag spinach

1. Wash spinach well—it's sandy. Set aside.
2. Wash and slice mushrooms. Set aside.
3. Diagonal-slice asparagus. Set aside.
4. Heat wok.
5. Necklace with oil.
6. Add asparagus and mushrooms. Stir fry.
7. Add all other ingredients.
8. Cover and steam, stirring occasionally.
9. Serve when veggies are crisp-tender.
10. Enjoy a very low-calorie, very filling meal.

SERVES 2

FLO AND EDDIE'S SESAME MUSHROOMS

When I was a very little girl, I had a big cousin who lived in an apartment downstairs from us. She taught me all the things big girls know—fascinating things like how to make ponytails, what kind of saddle shoes to buy, and even how and when to smile at the boys. Everything she knew was so important, so grown-up and special. Once she even taught me how to *dry dishes;* I remember thinking how marvelous that was, what a great thing to know. Everyone said I looked like Florence, and I held that to my heart like a special blessing.

Those two little girls seem fixed in time to me, as though they still exist somewhere in Queens, giggling now at the grown-up ladies we've become. If they are watching, they must be so amazed that Florence has a real husband and real children and that Annette writes cookbooks in New York City.

Here we are, all these years later, and Flo is still teaching me things—like what she and Eddie do with mushrooms! I *still* think everything she knows is unique and special.

INGREDIENTS:

    1 pound mushrooms
    2 cloves garlic, finely minced
       sesame oil
1½ tablespoons lemon juice
       salt and pepper to taste
    3 tablespoons sesame seeds

1. Wash mushrooms, remove stems from caps, and slice both.
2. Heat wok.
3. Necklace with sesame oil.
4. Saute garlic for 5 minutes.
5. Add mushrooms, sesame seeds, lemon juice, and salt and pepper.
6. Mix well. Simmer 10 minutes longer and serve.

SERVES 2

SIMPLE STEAMED CABBAGE

INGREDIENTS:

1 cup shredded cabbage
  salt and pepper to taste
1 tablespoon oil
1 clove garlic, finely minced

1. Rinse cabbage and drain well. Set aside.
2. Heat wok and necklace with oil.
3. Add garlic, stir fry till golden.
4. Add cabbage, sprinkle with salt and pepper and toss to combine.
5. Stir fry till cabbage is crisp-tender.

SERVES 2

AUNT MARY'S LOVELY LIMAS

INGREDIENTS:

1 10-ounce box frozen lima beans
1 small onion, chopped
1 small can tomato sauce
  oil for cooking
  salt and pepper to taste
  pinch of oregano
  pinch of basil

1. Heat wok.
2. Necklace with oil.
3. Stir fry onion.
4. Boil water and cook limas according to directions.
5. Add sauce to onions in wok. Add seasonings and stir.
6. Simmer for 15 minutes.
7. Add limas to wok.
8. Simmer for 5 more minutes and serve.

SERVES 2

BROCCOLI LEAVES

My Grandmom cooked and ate everything, making terrific meals out of nothing. She taught my mother, and that's how a recipe for broccoli leaves came to appear on the next page. Personally, I always wondered if there was something to be done with all those leaves every time I threw them away. It was not until I was hunting out the recipes for this book that I thought to ask my mother. Now I wish I'd thought to ask ten years ago! They're delicious, low-calorie, and vitamin-packed.

INGREDIENTS:

broccoli leaves from 1 head
1 medium-sized potato, cubed
1 tablespoon olive oil
salt and pepper to taste
1 clove garlic, on toothpick
water

1. Boil 1 cup salted water in wok, then add leaves and garlic on toothpick.
2. Cover and simmer for 10 minutes or until tender.
3. Drain off water, leaving ½ cup.
4. Add 1 tablespoon oil, salt and pepper to taste, and cubed potato.
5. Cover and cook till potato is tender. Remove garlic. (It will be easy to find on the toothpick!)
6. Serve in bowl with broth.

SERVES 2

GRANDMA'S ELBOWS AND KIDNEY BEANS

This is another Italian treat from the old country. Grandma served kidney beans and elbows for lunch in Naples and kept right on serving it in the promised land.

INGREDIENTS:

- 1 can red kidney beans, drained and rinsed
- 1 clove garlic, on toothpick
- 1 stalk celery, chopped
  salt and pepper to taste
- 1 tablespoon olive oil
- 1 cup cooked elbow macaroni
- ½ cup water with 1 teaspoon salt added

1. Boil ½ cup salted water in wok. Add celery, garlic on toothpick, salt and pepper, oil; cook until tender over low heat. Then remove garlic on toothpick.
2. Add beans and heat through. Add cooked macaroni.
3. Serve with broth.

SERVES 2

GINA'S LUNCH ON THE GO

7

LUNCH ON THE GO

No need to succumb to pastrami on rye. Here are treats you can make at home, pack up, and take to work! Keep thinking of that beautiful body you are creating, and the extra effort will come easy.

UMA'S LUNCH ON THE GO

This section is filled with recipes from a terrific woman who has made a profession of making lunches for people. Uma works with Integral Yoga Natural Foods on 14th Street between 7th and 8th avenues in New York City and prepares all the salads and sandwiches that are sold there. People flock to the store at lunchtime because Uma's lunch is the best in town. She generously agreed to share her secrets with us, and I'd like to thank both her and my wonderful family of friends at Integral Yoga for all of their love and support.

TOFU SANDWICH SPREAD

This is my favorite sandwich filling in the world!

INGREDIENTS:

- 6 tofu cakes, drained and mashed
- ¼ cup tamari or soy sauce
- ¼ cup tahini (sesame paste)
- ⅛ cup lemon juice
- 3 scallions, chopped
- ¼ cup alfalfa sprouts
- ¼ cup carrots, shredded
- ¼ cup cabbage, shredded

1. Combine first 4 ingredients. Mash together with fork.
2. Mix in carrots, scallions and cabbage.
3. Spread on bread. Top sandwich with sprouts and serve.

MAKES ENOUGH FOR 4 SANDWICHES

3 BEAN SALAD

INGREDIENTS:

¼ pound soybeans
¼ pound kidney beans
1½ pounds string beans

1. Soak beans overnight and in the morning boil till tender (about 1 hour).
2. Let cool.
3. Steam string beans in wok and let cool.
4. Combine all beans and toss with dressing.*
5. Chill and serve.

SERVES 4-6

* For dressing, see Dressing for Veggie and Soybeans (p. 78).

HUMMOUS

INGREDIENTS:

- 1 pound chick peas
- 8 ounces lemon juice
- 6 cloves garlic, minced
- 1 teaspoon cayenne pepper, or to taste
- 1 tablespoon salt, or to taste
- 2 cups tahini (sesame paste)

1. Soak chick peas for 1 hour in hot water. Cook for 1 hour till soft, then drain.
2. Blend lemon juice, garlic, cayenne, and salt till smooth. Pour into jar.
3. Begin to blend chick peas with lemon juice mixture and tahini in batches.
4. Either serve with pita bread as a dip or spread on pita with sprouts and tomato topping as a sandwich.

SERVES 4-6

FRESH BROCCOLI SALAD

This is a fairly large party-size quantity but can easily be cut down to suit your needs.

INGREDIENTS:

  1 bunch broccoli flowerets; chopped stems
  1 cup tahini (sesame paste)
 12 ounces alfalfa sprouts
  4 ounces carrots, shredded
  4 ounces cabbage, shredded
    spike seasoning to taste (spike is a natural blend of herbs and spices)

1. Combine all ingredients.
2. Have a party with it!

COOL CHILI

INGREDIENTS:

½ pound kidney beans, cooked according to instructions on package
3 small or 2 medium onions, chopped
2 green peppers, sliced
1 6-ounce can tomato paste mixed with 6 ounces water
2 cloves garlic
½ teaspoon chili powder or cayenne pepper
2 cups bulgur
4 cups water
2–3 teaspoons oregano
2–3 teaspoons salt
1 bay leaf
¼ teaspoon thyme
   oil for cooking

1. Heat wok.
2. Necklace with oil.
3. Stir fry pepper and onion till tender.
4. Add to beans in big bowl with rest of ingredients.
5. Refrigerate several hours and serve.

YIELD IS A WOKFUL!

VEGGIES AND SOYBEANS

INGREDIENTS:

½ pound cooked soybeans, drained and chilled
1 cucumber, sliced thinly
1 medium onion, diced
1 green pepper, diced
3 carrots, shredded
1 cup cabbage, shredded
1 cup broccoli, chopped

1. Combine all veggies.
2. Toss with dressing.
3. Chill and serve.

DRESSING:

¼ cup apple cider vinegar
2 cloves garlic
½ cup olive oil
  sea salt to taste
  pinch of oregano

1. Blend ingredients at high speed in electric blender.
2. Refrigerate till needed.

SERVES 4

COLE SLAW

For lunch or on the party buffet, a fresh cole slaw can't be beat!

INGREDIENTS:

1 head cabbage, shredded
1 pound carrots, shredded
1 small onion, chopped
1 green pepper, diced
6 ounces mayonnaise
    dash (generous) of cider vinegar
    sea salt to taste

1. Combine all ingredients.
2. Chill and serve.

SERVES 4-6 AS A SIDE DISH

UMA'S WHOLE-WHEAT BREAD

Because I know that at least *once* in a great while you are going to insist on some bread, I am including bread to die for. It is the most delicious and nutritional bread imaginable. Go easy. Bread is fat food—let a little go a long way and savor every speck of it.

INGREDIENTS:

⅓ cup safflower oil
3 cups hot water
3 teaspoons sea salt, dissolved
⅓ cup honey
⅓ cup raw millet
1 cup sunflower seeds
½ cup sesame seeds
1 cup currants (or raisins)
10–11 cups whole-wheat flour
1 tablespoon dry yeast in ½ cup lukewarm water (set aside)

1. Mix first 4 ingredients in big bowl.
2. Add next 4 and stir again.
3. Add yeast to above mixture.
4. Add whole-wheat flour until you can't stir any more—about 10 to 11 cups.
5. Knead until you're tired.
6. Let rise, punch down.
7. Place in 3 large, oiled loaf pans, and let rise again.
8. Bake in preheated oven at 400° F. for 10 minutes, then lower heat to 350° and bake for 40 more minutes.

Note: Add small pan of water in oven to keep bread moist.

YIELDS 3 LARGE LOAVES

TABOULI SALAD

Once you discover Tabouli Salad, it's a hard thing not to always have in your refrigerator. It's so easy and so good. It's made primarily from bulgur wheat, which is sold in natural food stores everywhere and costs about 55 cents a pound. That one pound will make two good-sized bowls of Tabouli. It's a perfect thing to take to work for lunch. It's also great as a substitute for cole slaw or potato salad at picnics, or all by itself as a light, nutritional meal. My gourmet friend Russell tells me he serves it hot, accompanying a main dinner course.

However you like it served, you'll probably consider Tabouli a diet food discovery of the decade!

INGREDIENTS:

       1 cup bulgur wheat
    1¾ cups water
       2 scallions
         juice of 1 lemon
       1 tomato
       1 cucumber
      ½ bunch fresh parsley
      ½ bunch fresh dill
       1 teaspoon sesame seeds (toasted first)
    1-2 tablespoons tamari or soy sauce
         oil (sesame is especially great here)
         salt and pepper to taste
         optional: a few leaves of fresh spearmint if you have it taste great.

1. Boil 1¾ cups water.
2. Heat wok.
3. Necklace with oil, then lower heat.
4. Add bulgur and gently saute.
5. When water comes to a boil, add water to wok. Turn off heat.
6. In 1 hour, all water should be absorbed. Pour off any that's left.
7. Meanwhile, chop scallions. Put in bowl.
8. Chop tomato and slice cucumber. Add to bowl.
9. Chop parsley and dill (also spearmint, if using). Add to bowl.
10. Add ingredients in bowl to bulgur in wok and toss.

11. Add tamari, sesame seeds, a little salt and pepper, and about 1 tea-spoon oil.
12. Squeeze in lemon juice and mix well.
13. Serve warm or refrigerate and serve as salad.

SERVES 4

FOR SHRIMP IN OYSTER SAUCE

8

DYNAMITE DINNERS

As simple or exotic as you choose

Imagine dinners so easy to make that in 15 minutes you can whip up a feast. Well, that's what's waiting for you in this chapter—healthy, beautiful dinners that will make cooking a simple pleasure and cleaning up a breeze.

I have included seafood, vegetables, and poultry and have eliminated red meat. As previously mentioned, red meat is very high in calories and difficult for your system to digest. As you wok your way skinny, I would suggest limiting your intake, perhaps enjoying a steak or whatever your favorite meat dish is as an occasional treat instead of the integral protein source in your diet. Protein is readily available in seafood, poultry, tofu, beans, nuts, seeds, and cheese. All contain much less bulk and are far less fattening.

TOFU SHRIMP IN OYSTER SAUCE

INGREDIENTS:

1 clove garlic
1 pound fresh shrimp, shelled, or frozen shrimp, defrosted
½ pound fresh, or 1 package frozen and defrosted, snow peas
1 cake bean curd
1 small onion
2 tablespoons oyster sauce (sold bottled in most grocery stores these days)
salt and pepper to taste
oil for cooking

1. Mince garlic and set aside.
2. If snow peas are fresh, wash and remove stems. Set aside.
3. Slice onion. Set aside.
4. Cut tofu into 1-inch pieces. Set aside.
5. Heat wok.
6. Necklace with oil.
7. Add garlic and onion. Stir fry till lightly golden.
8. Add shrimp. Stir fry for 1 minute.
9. Add tofu and snow peas. Stir fry till shrimp are pink.
10. Add oyster sauce, and salt and pepper to taste.
11. Simmer for 2 to 3 minutes and serve.

SERVES 2

BACKYARD CAULIFLOWER

At the completion of my last book, it was time to take some pictures. Steve Yaeger, a film director and photographer, flew up from Baltimore and started clicking away. We took pictures all over Fire Island and during a party that featured lots of wokked goodies and a tempura bar. Needless to say, after all this I was pretty cooked out!

The day after the party, I couldn't even *look* at food till late afternoon, when, at my mere *mention* of hunger, I was suddenly surrounded by friendly, hungry faces with gleaming eyes.

"Annette," they said, "we forgot pictures of wok barbecuing!"

They knew they had me. I crawled into the kitchen, and with party leftovers created a meal we liked so much we've all made it again and again. In retrospect, it was actually worth getting up for!

We made it over the barbecue coals. You can make it right over the stove as well.

INGREDIENTS:

- 1 head cauliflower
- 2 tomatoes
- ½ bunch fresh parsley
- 1 scallion
- 1 cup (approximately) of leftover brown rice
- ¾ cup sharp cheddar cheese, shredded
  tamari or soy sauce, to taste
  salt and pepper to taste
- ¼ teaspoon oregano
  oil for cooking

1. Break cauliflower into flowerets. Wash and slice into thin pieces.
2. Chop tomatoes into chunks.
3. Chop parsley and scallion.
4. Shred cheese. Set aside.
5. Heat wok.
6. Necklace with oil.
7. Add cauliflower. Stir fry for 2 to 3 minutes. Sprinkle a little cold water around sides of wok to create steam and cover for 3 to 5 minutes, stirring occasionally.
8. Add tomatoes, parsley, and scallion. Sprinkle with oregano and salt and pepper. Stir fry.

9. When vegetables are crisp-tender, add rice and tamari and stir fry till heated.

10. Sprinkle with cheese. Sprinkle sides of wok with water to create steam. Cover. When cheese is melted—FEAST!

SERVES 2

LADY A'S BLUE PLATE SPECIAL

Every cook has an old standby, a familiar-friend recipe that's a pleasure to fall back on. This one has become mine. I eat it often and with countless variations. It never disappoints—it's always inexpensive, easy, and delicious.

INGREDIENTS:

¾ cup walnut pieces
4 cups cooked rice (preferably cold)
3 carrots, shredded
1 head broccoli or cauliflower, finely chopped
2 medium-sized onions, minced
4 large mushrooms, sliced
  tamari to taste
1 tablespoon sesame seeds, toasted
  oil for cooking

1. Prepare all the veggies.
2. Heat wok.
3. Necklace with oil.
4. Add veggies and stir fry till almost tender.
5. Add rice and nuts and sprinkle with tamari. Stir well.
6. Add sesame seeds.
7. Stir till rice is heated and then serve.

Note: Variations can include fresh chopped ginger, tofu, and any assortment of available seasonal vegetables.

SERVES 2

CLUB MED'S PASTA PRIMAVERA

In Fire Island all the houses have names instead of numbers—"Sunset House," "Spot," "Act II," "Bottles Up." Well, our house was called "Club Med," because of the athletic interests that dominated its members. With my yoga instruction, Paul's gymnastics, Marc's running, Tom's boating, Arnie's and John's weightlifting, Steve's and Sue's swimming, Bill's fishing, Rene's and Laura's cycling and Ellen's and Margaret's exercises, it was a Club Med atmosphere indeed.

Our very favorite of all the recipes we shared that summer was this next one, Club Med's Pasta Primavera. It is a natural Italian delight. By using good whole grain pasta and lots of vegetables, the calorie count is down and the nutritional value up. It's our pleasure to share our specialty of the house, Club Med's Pasta Primavera!

INGREDIENTS:

1 pound whole grain pasta (spinach, whole-wheat, egg, or a combination)
2 cakes tofu, cubed
1 head broccoli, sliced
1 bunch scallions, chopped
1 clove garlic, minced
1 dozen cherry tomatoes
1 zucchini, sliced thinly
1 cup Parmesan cheese
½ cup milk
½ stick butter
oil for cooking
salt and pepper to taste
pinch of basil
pinch of oregano

1. Boil water for pasta and cook according to directions.
2. Heat wok.
3. Necklace with oil.
4. Add garlic and scallions. Stir fry till golden and remove to plate.
5. Stir fry broccoli in two batches and remove to plate.
6. Add zucchini and stir fry in two batches till crisp and golden. Add more oil if necessary.

7. Put all veggies back in wok. Add basil, oregano and salt and pepper to taste.
8. Add tofu and tomatoes and toss.
9. Drain pasta. When ready, place in a large bowl. Add butter, milk, and cheese. Toss well.
10. Place a portion of pasta in center of each plate. Ladle veggies on top, sprinkle with Parmesan cheese, and serve.

SERVES **4**

PASTA WITH PESTO AND TURKEY

INGREDIENTS:

oil for cooking
¼ pound mushrooms, thinly sliced
1 pound boneless turkey breast (or chicken), sliced paper thin
2 large scallions, thinly sliced on diagonal
¼ cup dry white wine
¾–1 pound pasta (short or long)
½ cup pesto (see page 91) diluted with ¼ cup pasta cooking water

1. Heat wok over high heat and necklace with oil.
2. Add mushrooms and stir fry for 1 to 2 minutes until mushrooms are browned and begin to release the oil they soaked up.
3. Add turkey and stir fry for 1 to 2 minutes until turkey is no longer pink.
4. Add scallions and stir fry briefly.
5. Add wine, cover wok, and steam for 1 minute. Turn off heat.
6. Cook pasta (3 ounces per serving, or more if you've done your exercises today) in 5 quarts of boiling, salted water until done *al dente*.
7. Just before pasta is done, ladle off ¼ cup of the cooking water and mix it with the pesto. When pasta is done, drain well but do not rinse.
8. Place pasta in large, warmed serving bowl. Pour pesto over it and toss well. Add turkey mixture and toss again.

SERVES 4

SKIP'S PESTO

INGREDIENTS:

¼ pound fresh basil (6 cups loosely packed leaves)
½ cup chopped walnuts
½ cup chopped parsley (firmly packed)
1 cup grated Parmesan
3–4 tablespoons garlic, minced (or to taste)
2 teaspoons coarsely ground pepper (or to taste)
¾ cup olive oil

1. Rinse basil well (it's often sandy) and drain well in colander.
2. If you have a food processor, you can do this in one batch; if you're using a blender, do it in three batches. Place all ingredients except oil in bowl of processor fitted with steel blade (or ⅓ of each ingredient except oil in blender container). Process or blend until almost a puree. With processor or blender running, add oil in a continuous stream until all of it is incorporated (for blender add ⅓ of the oil to each batch).
3. Store pesto in an airtight container. Keeps in the refrigerator for about a week. Freezes excellently. (I freeze it in 1-cup containers.) Remove from freezer and let thaw at room temperature until it's just soft enough to spoon out the desired amount. Return the rest to the freezer immediately. Makes an excellent sauce for pasta, vegetables, poultry, fish. Or for a green salad, mix 1 tablespoon pesto with 1 tablespoon fresh lemon juice or dry white wine per serving.

MAKES ABOUT 2¼ CUPS

TOFU PARMIGIANA

INGREDIENTS:

oil for cooking
1½ pounds tofu (see note on tofu, page 46)
 2 eggs
 1 tablespoon tamari or soy sauce
 ¾ cup wheat germ or bran (bran is less fattening)
 ¾ cup grated Parmesan
 ½ cup onions, sliced
 1 carrot, shredded
 2 cloves garlic, minced (or to taste)
 1 cup mushrooms, sliced
 2 cups tomatoes, seeded and diced (or 1 cup thick puree)
 1 tablespoon fresh basil, chopped (or 1 teaspoon dried)
 1 teaspoon oregano
 ¼ teaspoon crushed red pepper
sea salt to taste
 8 thin slices mozzarella (low fat)
cooked brown rice

1. Slice tofu cakes into 8 thin and equal slices.
2. In a shallow bowl, beat the eggs with the tamari until frothy and well blended.
3. Mix together wheat germ (or bran) and ¼ cup of the Parmesan on a dinner plate or pie plate.
4. Dip each tofu slice in egg, then in wheat germ and Parmesan mixture so that it is completely coated. Place coated tofu slices on a plate in single layer and refrigerate while you prepare sauce.
5. Heat wok over high heat and necklace with oil.
6. Add onions, carrot, garlic, and mushrooms and stir fry for several minutes until onions are translucent.
7. Add tomatoes, basil, oregano, and red pepper. Stir well, bring to the boil, reduce heat, and simmer (not boil) uncovered for 15 to 20 minutes or until vegetables are soft.
8. When sauce is done, add salt to taste. Transfer to bowl and set aside.
9. Wipe out wok. Heat clean wok over high heat and necklace with oil.
10. Fry sliced tofu two or three at a time, turning once, until golden.
11. Heat broiler. Cover bottom of shallow rectangular baking pan with a thin layer of sauce and sprinkle with ¼ cup of the Parmesan.

Place browned tofu slices on sauce in a single layer. Top each tofu slice with a thin slice of mozzarella. Pour remaining sauce over and around tofu. Sprinkle remaining Parmesan over all.

12. Place under hot broiler until top is bubbly and beginning to brown and mozzarella is melted. Serve with cooked brown rice.

SERVES 4

LETTUCE-WRAPPED FLOUNDER FILLETS WITH SAVORY MUSHROOM FILLING

INGREDIENTS:

4 heads Boston or bibb lettuce (pick the largest heads you can find)
2 teaspoons tahini (sesame paste)
1 pound flounder fillet, cut in 4 equal oblong or rectangular portions
2 tablespoons butter
3 large scallions, finely minced
1 clove garlic, finely minced
¾ pound mushrooms, finely chopped
¼ cup fresh lemon juice
¼ cup parsley, finely chopped
½ cup cooked brown rice
½ teaspoon freshly ground pepper
½ cup dry white wine
1 cup plain yogurt (optional)

1. Place whole lettuce heads in wok or large kettle. Cover with boiling water and simmer for 1 minute to soften lettuce. Remove lettuce from simmering water and drain upside down in a colander.
2. Rub one side of each flounder fillet with ½ teaspoon of the tahini paste. Set fillets aside.
3. Dry wok if you used it to braise lettuce. Place 2 tablespoons butter in wok and heat over medium heat until butter has melted and is bubbly. Be careful not to burn butter.
4. Add half of the scallions and all of the garlic. Stir fry for 1 minute.
5. Turn heat to high. Add mushrooms and stir fry for several minutes until mushrooms have begun to exude their juices.
6. Add lemon juice to mushrooms and stir fry briskly until most of liquid has evaporated. The mixture should be thick and dark, not soupy.
7. Turn off heat. Add parsley, rice, and pepper to mushroom mixture and toss to combine ingredients.
8. Place 1 or 2 tablespoons of the mushroom mixture in the center of the tahini-coated side of each flounder fillet. Fold the 2 longer ends of the fillet up and over the stuffing, so that each fillet becomes an open-ended roll.

9. Pick off 16 of the largest lettuce leaves. You will use 4 for each fillet. Make a four-leaf clover design with 4 lettuce leaves but with the stem ends pointing out instead of touching each other. Allow the leafy ends of the lettuce to overlap each other. If the 4 leaves are not large enough to overlap each other, use some of the remaining smaller leaves to fill in the gaps.

10. Place a rolled fillet in the center of the lettuce leaf arrangement. Completely wrap the fillet by folding the stem ends of the lettuce leaves one at a time up and over the fillet. Repeat with the remaining fillets and large lettuce leaves.

11. Remove any leftover mushroom mixture from the wok. Reserve for another use. (It makes a delicious filling for an omelet.)

12. Line bottom of wok with any remaining lettuce leaves. Sprinkle 1 large, finely minced scallion over leaves. Carefully place lettuce-wrapped fillets stem side down in wok.

13. Pour white wine over fillets. Turn heat to medium, cover tightly, and bring to the simmer. Simmer very gently (DO NOT BOIL) for 15 minutes.

14. Carefully remove wrapped fillets and lettuce leaves that lined bottom of wok to a warmed serving platter. Cover and keep warm.

15. Boil liquid remaining in wok over high heat until reduced in volume by half. Spoon reduced liquid over wrapped fillets and serve with brown rice OR ...

16. Reduce liquid by half as in Step 15. Turn heat to low, stir in 1 cup yogurt and heat through but do not boil. Pour into a warmed bowl or sauceboat and let each of your guests spoon out the sauce as desired.

SERVES 4

CHICKEN SUZANNE

Career people working in New York City are incredibly busy. The competition is stiff, so the hours are long and sometimes it's hard to have time for basic survival. My friend Suzanne Lobel, an art director at Zebra Books in Manhattan, told me that without a wok, she wouldn't be able to cope with cooking dinner at night and would never manage to keep her tall, trim body in shape. This next recipe is one she says she eats all the time—her old standby both for a quick meal alone or when company's coming!

INGREDIENTS:

½ pound mushrooms, sliced
½ pound snow peas, with ends clipped
1 bunch broccoli
1 can water chestnuts, drained and sliced
1 red pepper, sliced into thin strips
1 green pepper, sliced into thin strips
4 chicken breasts, cut into chunks
3 carrots, sliced diagonally
4 scallions, chopped
1 tablespoon sesame seeds
1 garlic clove
  salt and pepper to taste
6 thin slices ginger, chopped very fine
  tamari or soy sauce, to taste
  oil for cooking
  cooked brown rice

1. Rub wok with garlic.
2. Heat wok.
3. Necklace with oil.
4. Sprinkle chicken chunks with tamari, and add chunks to wok.
5. Stir fry till chicken is white, then remove to plate.
6. Add carrots and broccoli to wok. Cook till almost tender.
7. Add ginger plus all other vegetables except snow peas. Stir fry.
8. Put chicken back in wok. Stir.
9. Add snow peas. Stir.
10. Season with additional tamari and salt and pepper to taste.
11. Sprinkle with sesame seeds and serve over rice.

SERVES 4

CRAB OR CHICKEN DIVAN

When the word went out that I was collecting new recipes for another book, I was pleasantly surprised with a contribution from a "Re-Form School For The Overweight" in California.

Thanks, Connie Levy! And thanks, Barbara Tint, for putting us in touch.

INGREDIENTS:

    12 ounces crab or chicken (cooked)
1½–2 pounds broccoli, cut into thin flowerets
    2 tablespoons flour
    ½ cup nonfat milk
    2 ounces mozzarella cheese
    1 teaspoon salt
    ¼ teaspoon pepper
    1 16-ounce can tomatoes
      pinch of paprika
      oil for cooking

1. Heat wok.
2. Necklace with oil.
3. Stir fry broccoli for 3 minutes or until almost tender and place in bottom of baking dish.
4. Cut crab or chicken into bite-size pieces and arrange over broccoli.
5. Put flour, salt, and pepper in wok over low heat, and add milk, stirring constantly until thick.
6. Add the cheese and stir till blended, then add tomatoes.
7. Pour mixture over the crab or chicken. Sprinkle with paprika. Bake at 400° F. for 15 minutes or until browned.

SERVES 4

SWEET NAOMI'S COCONUT COGNAC CHICKEN

People familiar with Fire Island are very often familiar with "Sweet Naomi's Goodies"—a line of delicious, natural baked goods that provide a healthy alternative to the usual sugar-filled desserts available. Naomi's awareness of healthy cooking continues into her main course creations, as you will discover in the following recipe: her yummy Coconut Cognac Chicken that features coconut, apples, and walnuts!

INGREDIENTS:

2 cups chicken, cut into thin slices
1 green apple, chopped
3 tablespoons shredded coconut
1 cup chopped walnuts
   oil for cooking
2 tablespoons chicken stock or water
1 tablespoon cognac
1 tablespoon Hoisin sauce
1 teaspoon tamari or soy sauce
   cooked brown rice

1. Heat wok.
2. Necklace with oil.
3. Add chicken. Stir fry till chicken is white, then remove to plate.
4. Add to wok apple, coconut, walnuts, and stock. Stir fry for 3 minutes or until apple is nearly tender.
5. Put chicken back in wok. Add cognac, Hoisin sauce, and tamari. Heat through and serve over rice.

SERVES 2

HONEY SESAME CHICKEN

What a great diet! You can even use a little honey on your way to being skinny!

This was a spontaneous invention that my friend Brian and I liked so much it became our favorite glaze for chicken. You can even use it for flavoring broiled or roasted chicken. The combination is finger-licking good!

INGREDIENTS:

- 1 tablespoon honey
- 1 teaspoon sesame oil
- 1 teaspoon sesame seeds
- 2 boneless breasts of chicken
- 1 fresh tomato
- 1 small onion
- 6–8 asparagus stalks if in season, or 1 small head broccoli
- tamari or soy sauce, to taste
- salt and pepper to taste
- ¼ teaspoon oregano
- ¼ teaspoon dried or 1 teaspoon fresh basil
- oil for cooking

1. Combine honey and sesame oil. Mix well to form paste.
2. With your fingers, rub paste onto chicken breasts. Set aside.
3. Cut tomato into large chunks. Set aside.
4. Slice onion. Set aside.
5. Diagonally slice asparagus or broccoli into thin pieces. Set aside.
6. Slice chicken breasts into ½-inch strips.
7. Heat wok.
8. Necklace with oil.
9. Add chicken a few pieces at a time and stir fry, sprinkling each batch with sesame seeds and salt and pepper. Remove to plate.
10. Add onion to wok (adding a drop more oil if necessary). Stir fry for 1 to 2 minutes.
11. Add tomato and season with oregano and basil.
12. Add sliced asparagus or broccoli and stir fry till vegetables are crisp-tender.
13. Return chicken to wok.
14. Add tamari to taste.
15. Simmer a moment more and serve.

SERVES 2

ANTOINETTE'S CHICKEN CAPONATA

INGREDIENTS:

1½ pounds chicken parts
  2 cups caponata (see page 59)
    oil for cooking

1. Heat wok.
2. Necklace with oil.
3. Brown the chicken parts a few at a time.
4. Place all back in wok.
5. Add caponata.
6. Lower heat and cover. Simmer for 20 minutes or until chicken is tender.

SERVES 2

NO-SWEAT SEVICHE AND RICE SALAD

A fine, somewhat unusual preparation of seafood is done by cooking with citric acid instead of heat.

We use that process in this next recipe. By marinating the scallops or whitefish fillets in lime juice for several hours, we never need to use heat. Once the fish has turned completely white and the texture is firm, you know it's ready.

INGREDIENTS:

- 1 pound bay scallops, sea scallops, or firm-fleshed white fish (cod, flounder, sole, halibut)
- ⅓ cup freshly squeezed lime or lemon juice
- 1 clove garlic, minced
- 3 large scallions, thinly sliced
- 1 medium Italian sweet green pepper, cored, seeded, and coarsely chopped
- 1 small hot green pepper, cored, seeded, finely minced (optional)
- 1 cup tomato, coarsely chopped
- ¼ cup freshly snipped dill (or 2 teaspoons dried)
- ¼ cup parsley, minced
- 2 cups fresh mung bean sprouts, well drained
- 2 cups cooked brown rice, cooled
- 1 tablespoon tamari or soy sauce
  hot chili oil or Tabasco to taste (if you haven't used hot green pepper)

1. If you are using sea scallops or whitefish, cut into bite-size pieces. Combine scallops or fish, lime juice, 1 of the sliced scallions, and garlic in a stainless steel, glass, or ceramic bowl. Toss well, making sure seafood is coated with lime juice. Cover and refrigerate for several hours. Stir occasionally.
2. When seafood is "cooked," drain off and reserve ½ cup of marinade.
3. In large serving bowl, combine remaining ingredients except reserved marinade, tamari, and hot pepper or hot chili oil.
4. Combine reserved marinade with tamari and pepper or chili oil. Sprinkle over salad, toss, and serve.

SERVES 2

BABY'S BUTTERNUT STEW

Named in honor of their baby on the way . . . another treat from John and Annie.

INGREDIENTS:

1 clove garlic, minced
1 butternut squash, seeded and cut into large chunks with peel on
1 onion, cut into large chunks
2 carrots, cut in chunks
¼ cup water
½ teaspoon thyme
olive oil for cooking
1 head broccoli, separated into flowerets and stems sliced
1 tablespoon Genmai Miso* diluted with 3 tablespoons water, or tamari or soy sauce, to taste

1. Heat wok.
2. Necklace with oil.
3. Stir fry squash, onion, and garlic till golden brown.
4. Add carrots, ¼ cup water, and thyme and cover. Simmer till almost tender.
5. Add broccoli. Add small amount of water if needed. When broccoli is tender, turn off heat.
6. Add miso mixture or tamari and toss. Let sit for 5 minutes and serve. It's great over whole-wheat noodles!

SERVES 2

* Genmai Miso is a variety of miso paste and can be found in your natural food store.

RICHIE'S BLACKFISH

Stalking the seas of Fire Island is a spear fisherman that has even the blackfish running scared. Richie Covello introduced me to what was to become the highlight of my summer season—spear fishing. For the past 15 years, instead of using a rod and reel, Richie has been using only his wits and his spear to bring home dinner. I watched from a boat once and knew the next time out I wanted to be dressed in a wet suit and be part of the action. What a sport! My first day out in a wet suit was Test Day. From his perch on the Kismet pier, Richie had me snorkel, dive, do breath checks, and swim distance. When I satisfied him that I was comfortable and confident in the water, we began the swim out. As most of Kismet sipped drinks on the shore during Happy Hour, we made our way out into the channel. My first real dive convinced me I would be enjoying skin diving for a long time to come. It brought me into a school of blackfish. These are big fish—ranging from 15 to 40 pounds! We swam over reefs and sunken ships and I became part of a bay that before had been something to merely ferry across! Once in the water, I realized we literally became part of the food chain as we watched for sharks and the blackfish watched for us. Luckily, we came out ahead that time, securing a 15-pound black for supper. Tired but exhilarated, we emerged at the pier sometime later with dinner over our shoulders and the wet suits peeled to our skins. We came home and made what was to become known as Richie's Blackfish.

(Blackfish is not easily available commercially due to the difficulty in catching them: they're fighters. Flounder, sole, or trout can be substituted.)

INGREDIENTS:

- 4 large blackfish fillets (or other whitefish)
- ½ cup chopped scallions
- 1 tablespoon lemon juice
- 1 cup white wine
- ¼ cup parsley, finely minced
- 1 teaspoon sesame oil
- 1 teaspoon sesame seeds
- boiling water
- cooked brown rice

1. Place boiling water in wok.
2. Place steam rack in wok.

3. Arrange fillets in heat-proof serving dish.
4. Pour wine and lemon juice over fillets.
5. Sprinkle with chopped scallions, parsley, and sesame seeds.
6. Drizzle with sesame oil.
7. Cover and allow to steam in wok for 15 to 20 minutes, or until fish flakes easily with fork.
8. Serve with brown rice.

SERVES 4

SPRING STREET NATURAL*

One of the most popular recipes in my first wok cookbook came from the kitchen of one of the finest natural restaurants in New York City—Spring St. Natural. Nestled in Soho, it's an absolute delight to visit. From homemade soups to unique salads, fabulous entrees, and luscious desserts, Spring St. Natural remains one of my very favorite places in the world. Along with wonderful food and ambiance, the quality of the people is top notch. Owner Robert Schoenholt, manager Eric Eloenhorn, and headwaitress Elaine team up to make sure all their customers have a perfect time. A recipe from them is a gourmet treat, and here it comes . . .

* Spring St. Natural, 149 Spring Street, New York City, (212) 966-0290.

SPRING STREET NATURAL'S FILLET OF SOLE WITH RED AND BLACK GINGER SAUCE

To steam fish:

Place 1½–2 pounds fillet of sole on lightly oiled round platter; place platter on steam rack in wok. Put boiling water beneath rack, cover, and steam for 20 minutes or until sole flakes with fork.

Red Sauce:
INGREDIENTS:

> ½ cup Chinese pickled red ginger, cut julienne (reserve juice)
> 1½ cups water
> 1 tablespoon brown sugar
> ¼ cup rice vinegar
> 1 teaspoon cornstarch mixed in 2 tablespoons cold water
>   salt to taste

1. Combine first four ingedients with wire whisk over low heat in saucepan.
2. Bring to boil. Add cornstarch/water mixture. Lower heat and simmer till needed.

Black Sauce:
INGREDIENTS:

> ½ cup tamari or soy sauce
> 1 teaspoon garlic, minced
> 1 teaspoon fresh ginger, minced
>   juice of ½ lemon
> 1½ cups water
> ¼ cup Shao Hsing wine or dry sherry
> 1½ tablespoons cornstarch mixed in 2 tablespoons cold water

1. Combine all ingredients in saucepan.
2. Bring to boil.
3. Strain and bring back to boil.
4. Whisk in cornstarch.
5. Simmer till needed.

To serve:

1. Take platter from wok when fish is ready.
2. Pour Red Sauce over half the fillets.
3. Pour Black Sauce over other half.
4. Garnish with chopped scallions.

SERVES **4**

EDDIE AND EILEEN'S WALNUT TARRAGON CHICKEN

If I had to pick a couple to be stranded with anywhere in the world, I would pick Eddie and Eileen Friedman. The primary reason is because wherever they are, they always have a great time. They are one of those blessed couples who maintain their sense of fun and good humor throughout all of life's changing scenes, and who are genuinely interested in everything there is to learn. When we met, food was an insignificant part of their lifestyle. They worked incredibly long hours at their film-editing company—DJM—all week long and on the weekends they played hard on their beautiful boat—*Eddie's Mink*. Well, after a few outings together on the boat, Eileen and Eddie agreed to experiment: instead of preparing the regular deck barbecue, we tried out wokked food to see how it went over with family and friends. As usual, people flipped over the fare and Eileen could not believe how easy it was to prepare. That was it. The next step was turning their townhouse kitchen into a real Wokmaster's studio. I called First Stop Housewares, my favorite houseware store on 2nd Ave. at 54th St. in New York City, and had them deliver everything from a rice pot to a cutting board—all that she would need.

Well, Eileen's a bona fide Wokmaster now. In fact, her diet is exclusively wok food and sushi and her body never looked better. Eddie says both the food and the figure have won his heart. As a very special thank you for all the wonderful fun we've had together, I've created this next dish in their honor.

INGREDIENTS:

½ cup walnuts
2 boneless breasts of chicken, diced (about 2 lbs.)
2 scallions, chopped
½ teaspoon tarragon
2 carrots, sliced finely
2 tablespoons apple cider vinegar or to taste
cooked brown rice
oil for cooking

1. Heat wok.
2. Necklace with oil.
3. Stir fry chicken with tarragon and walnuts till chicken is white. Remove to plate.

4. Add scallions and carrots to wok. Stir fry till crisp-tender.
5. Add tarragon and chicken and walnuts to vegetables in wok. Stir together.
6. Splash with vinegar. Stir and serve over rice.

SERVES 4

SUSAN'S SWEET AND SOUR CHICKEN

Also from the office of DJM comes a new Wokmaster's creation. Susan invented a delicious sweet and sour chicken dish. Enjoy!

INGREDIENTS:

2 chicken breasts, cubed (about 2 lbs.)
2 stalks celery, sliced
1 green pepper, sliced
1 can water chestnuts, sliced
2 scallions, chopped
1 package frozen or 8 ounces fresh snow peas
1 can pineapple (drain and reserve juice)

Sauce:

¼ cup dry white wine
¼ cup honey
2 tablespoons cornstarch, diluted in juice from can of pineapple
oil for cooking

1. Heat wok.
2. Necklace with oil.
3. Cook chicken till white and remove to plate.
4. Put in wok green pepper, scallions, and celery. Cook covered until tender (about 4 to 7 minutes).
5. Add water chestnuts, pineapple, and snow peas.
6. In a bowl mix sauce ingredients, add to mixture in wok, and simmer for 2 minutes. Serve over brown rice.

SERVES 4

COMBINATION VEGETABLE SEAFOOD TEMPURA

Tempura is a party, and also one of the best-tasting ways of preparing vegetables there is. It's also a lot easier to prepare than most people think. At my birthday party last year, I set up a "tempura bar" in the backyard that was tremendously successful. An oil-filled wok over hot coals was in the center of a table with a bowl of batter and a tray of cut-up fresh vegetables and tamari dip next to it. I started the cooking but soon let my friends take over. Everyone played chef with great pleasure and success.

This recipe is for a combination vegetable and seafood tempura, with a batter that is especially light and delicate. I'm including it as a party treat while you wok your way skinny.

INGREDIENTS:

An array of cut-up vegetables, shrimp, fish fillets, and tofu enough for as many people as you have
1. Cut cauliflower and broccoli into large flowerets.
2. Leave mushrooms whole.
3. Cut tofu into big 2-inch chunks.
4. Shell shrimp, leaving on tail. Slice up the back of the shrimp to fan it out and slash with small strikes on each side to prevent curling.
5. Slice fillets into 3-inch pieces.
6. Cut onions into thick rings.
7. Slice cucumber, zucchini, and carrots.
8. Cut eggplant into thick rings.

Tempura Batter

INGREDIENTS:

2 eggs
1 cup minus 1 tablespoon ice water
¾ cup flour (unbleached white)
½ teaspoon salt
    oil for cooking
    chopped parsley or dill (optional)

1. Beat the eggs with the ice water.
2. Add flour and salt and beat very lightly (too much beating will bring out the gluten in the flour and make the batter sticky).

3. The secret of tempura is very hot oil and *very* cold batter. Fill a large bowl with ice cubes and cold water and sit the batter bowl in it.
4. Heat wok filled ⅔ with oil.* It's ready at 375°F., 191°C.
5. Dip sliced fish and vegetables in batter and drop in hot oil.
6. Start with one or two slices in the wok. As oil gets very, very hot, more can be cooked at once.
7. Keep oven on a low heat and as the tempura is ready, place in pan on rack to keep warm.
8. Serve on a bed of lettuce with fresh lemon and a dip on the side.

Easy Tempura Dip

1. To ½ cup tamari or soy sauce add ¼ cup broth or water.
2. Add 2 tablespoons grated fresh ginger and 1 finely chopped scallion.
3. Store in refrigerator.

Tempura "Pine Needles" Decoration

1. Take 5 or 6 strands of thin spaghetti and break off 3-inch pieces.
2. Holding pieces tightly together, dip into batter about ¾ of an inch deep and then dip into oil, still holding the strands together at the top.
3. In about 1 minute, let go. The strands will spread out in a fan and can be used for decoration of tempura bowl.

* Oil can be strained and kept in the refrigerator for reuse.

RUSSELL BENNETT'S AVOCADO SCALLOPS AND MUSHROOM GRATINEE

Russell Bennett has been my friend and collaborator for as long as I have been in the food industry. My second book, *Recipe For A Great Affair—How To Cater Your Own Party Or Anybody Else's*, was co-authored by him. Since he is a well-known New York caterer, Russell's recipes are a very special addition to this collection.

Remember when I said in the beginning that you can have anything you want while you wok your way skinny? Well, here's the proof. Avocados and cheese are not exactly carrot sticks and cottage cheese! But with balanced eating, you can enjoy them—guilt-free!

INGREDIENTS:

- 1 ripe avocado
- 12 large fresh mushroom caps, destemmed
- ½ pound bay scallops
- juice of 1 lime
- juice of 1 lemon
- 1 teaspoon dry dill or 1 tablespoon fresh dill
- 1 teaspoon Dijon mustard
- 1 tablespoon peanut oil
- 1 cup (½ pound) shredded low-fat mozzarella
- ½ teaspoon lemon pepper

1. Rinse scallops. Necklace wok with oil. Stir fry scallops with dill, adding lime and lemon juice. Cook till opaque (about 2 minutes). Remove from wok and let cool.
2. Cut avocado into tiny cubes. Toss with scallops, adding mustard and lemon pepper.
3. Spoon scallop mixture into mushroom caps and top with cheese.
4. Arrange caps in cake rack and place back in wok. Add ½ cup water in bottom of wok for steam.
5. Bring water to boil. Place lid on wok and steam 2 minutes to melt cheese.
6. Serve!

SERVES 4

RUSSELL BENNETT'S TWIST OF LEMON CHICKEN

INGREDIENTS:

2 pounds boneless chicken breast
3 lemons (2 sliced into thin rounds, 1 for juice)
1 tablespoon dried parsley flakes or fresh parsley, finely chopped
1 small clove garlic, finely chopped
1 tablespoon oil
½ teaspoon fresh ground pepper

1. Cut chicken into small strips.
2. Necklace hot wok with oil, add chopped garlic, stir, and add thinly sliced lemon and chicken together.
3. While stir frying, add lemon juice, parsley, and pepper and continue cooking until chicken is done (about 4 minutes).
4. Remove from wok and serve.

SERVES 4-6

SKIP'S PASTA WITH WHITE CLAM AND MUSHROOM SAUCE

INGREDIENTS:

  2 tablespoons olive oil
  ½ pound mushrooms, thinly sliced
  3 large cloves of garlic, minced (or to taste)
  2 tablespoons fresh basil, minced (or 2 teaspoons dried)
  1 teaspoon oregano
  ¼ teaspoon dried crushed red pepper (or to taste)
  2 6½–7-ounce cans chopped or minced clams with liquid drained and reserved (buy clams with no preservatives)
    reserved clam juice plus enough dry white wine to make 2 cups liquid
  2 large scallions, thinly sliced on diagonal
  ¼ cup parsley, finely chopped
    freshly grated Parmesan
  ¾ pounds whole grain pasta

1. Heat wok over high heat and necklace with 2 tablespoons olive oil.
2. Add mushrooms and stir fry briskly until the liquid the mushrooms exude has evaporated.
3. Add garlic, basil, oregano, and crushed red pepper. Stir fry 1 minute.
4. Add the 2 cups clam juice/wine mixture. Bring to the boil and cook vigorously for 5 minutes.
5. Turn heat down to medium. Add drained clams, scallions, and parsley, and bring to the simmer. Cover and turn off heat.
6. Boil pasta in 6 quarts of water until *al dente*. Drain but do not rinse.
7. Transfer pasta to warmed serving bowl or platter. Pour sauce over pasta. Toss well.
8. Sprinkle with freshly grated Parmesan to taste. There is enough sauce for ¾–1 pound pasta.

SERVES 3–4

POACHED SALMON WITH YOGURT DILL SAUCE

INGREDIENTS:

    2 pound piece of fresh salmon, weighed before skinning and boning,
      or 4–5-ounce fillets (see note)
      cold water
    1 medium onion, peeled and quartered
    ½ cup carrots, scraped and sliced
    1 stalk of celery with leaves, sliced
  5–6 sprigs parsley
    1 bay leaf
    ½ teaspoon thyme
    ¼ cup white wine vinegar or fresh lemon juice
    ⅓ cup fresh dill, minced
    1 teaspoon Dijon-style mustard (or to taste)
    1 cup plain yogurt
      dill sprigs for garnish

1. Place filleted salmon, cut into 4 equal portions, in wok.
2. Add cold water to cover the salmon by ¾ of an inch. Add onion, carrots, celery, parsley, bay leaf, thyme, and white wine vinegar or lemon juice. Turn heat to medium and bring to the simmer. Cover and simmer gently over medium-low heat for 15 minutes. Turn heat off and let salmon sit in the broth for 5 minutes.
3. Carefully remove salmon to a warmed plate. Cover and keep warm.
4. With skimmer, remove vegetables from broth. (Save vegetables for your Garbage Bag Stock, page 122.)
5. Boil broth over high heat until reduced to ¾ of a cup.
6. Turn heat to low. Add dill and mustard.
7. Stir in yogurt. Heat through but do not boil.
8. Place salmon fillets on warmed plates. Spoon several tablespoons of sauce over each fillet. Garnish with a sprig of dill. Pass remaining sauce at the table.

Note: Don't attempt this dish if fresh salmon and fresh dill aren't available. Canned salmon and dried dill simply won't do. Poached salmon is delicious, elegant, and remarkably simple to prepare for a dinner party. Braised leeks and baked potatoes are perfect accompaniments.

SERVES **4**

CHICKEN BREASTS WITH WATERCRESS AND FETA STUFFING

INGREDIENTS:

- 2 whole boneless chicken breasts (about 2 pounds)
- 2 tablespoons fresh lemon juice
- 2 bunches watercress
  oil for cooking
- 4 ounces mushrooms, thinly sliced
- 2 large scallions, minced
- 1 clove garlic, minced
- ¼ teaspoon freshly ground pepper
- 2 ounces feta cheese, crumbled
- 1 cup tomato puree
- 2 tablespoons fresh basil, minced (or 2 teaspoons dried)
- 1 teaspoon oregano

1. Split chicken breasts in half down the breastbone line. Place each breast half between two sheets of waxed paper and pound with a meat mallet or heavy flat-bottomed mug as thin as possible without breaking the fiber of the meat. Rub both sides of each flattened breast half with fresh lemon juice and set aside.

2. Rinse watercress, shake off excess moisture, and strip leaves from stems. Reserve stems for your Garbage Bag Stock (page 122).

3. Heat wok over medium-high heat. Do not necklace with oil yet. Add watercress leaves and stir briskly until they wilt. You may want to use a wooden spoon for this, since the leaves are tiny and not easily managed with chopsticks.

4. When leaves are wilted (it won't take long) remove them from the wok and place them in a colander to drain and cool.

5. Wipe out wok. Heat cleaned wok over high heat and necklace with oil. Add sliced mushrooms and stir fry until moisture mushrooms give off has evaporated.

6. Add scallions and garlic to mushrooms and stir fry 1 minute. Turn heat down to low while you . . .

7. Take a handful of the cooled watercress leaves and squeeze gently to remove excess moisture. Add squeezed watercress to mushroom/scallion mixture in wok. Turn heat back up to high. Add

freshly ground pepper and stir fry 1 minute or until mixture is steaming. Turn off heat.

8. Place 1 tablespoon of the watercress/mushroom mixture in the center of each flattened breast half. Sprinkle 1 tablespoon of the crumbled feta on top of this and cover the feta with another tablespoon of the stuffing. (Depending on the size of the flattened breasts, you may have to use less or more than 2 tablespoons of the stuffing per breast half.)

9. Fold the edges of each breast up over the stuffing so that the stuffing is completely enclosed and makes a neat package. (This process is similar to closing the four top flaps of a cardboard carton, tucking the corner of the last fold under the corner of the first fold to secure it.)

10. Remove any leftover stuffing from the wok and reserve. Wipe out wok. Heat cleaned wok over medium-high heat and necklace with 1 teaspoon oil.

11. Place the stuffed breasts, folded sides down, carefully into wok. Cover wok and heat gently for about 5 minutes. You're not frying them but heating them through.

12. While the breasts are heating, place the tomato puree, basil, oregano, and any reserved stuffing in a small saucepan and bring to the simmer.

13. When the puree simmers, pour it gently over and around the breasts in the wok. Cover wok and simmer gently for 15 minutes or until breasts are cooked. (The breasts are done when they feel springy rather than soft when pressed with a finger.)

14. With a spatula, carefully remove the breasts from the wok. Serve on a bed of pasta or with your favorite grain on warmed plates. Spoon sauce over breasts. Sprinkle with the rest of the crumbled feta.

Note: An interesting note about watercress is that *all* watercress is organic. It grows in water and it won't grow if there are any impurities present.

SERVES 4

BRUCE'S WOK LOBSTER

Imagine a man as good in the kitchen as he is on Wall Street and you will have begun to imagine Bruce Dorfman.

Bruce is a Wall Street economic consultant and the author, along with Ira Cobleigh, of *The Dowbeaters* and *The Roaring '80's On Wall Street* (Macmillan). We met at a party sometime back when in the midst of casual party talk both of us admitted to being in the crazy final week of closing out our second books. The week before a manuscript is due is usually filled with rewrites, research, typists, and editors. Our first "date" was hardly a social affair, as we sat in my living room with thousands of sheets of paper around us bouncing ideas off each other and rather frantically preparing the final manuscripts for submission. Well, the books turned out great—and so did we. I learned an enormous amount about Wall Street—and Bruce became a Wokmaster!

INGREDIENTS:

2–3 cups raw lobster meat pieces (either fresh, canned, or frozen; if using frozen lobster tails, figure 2 small tails per person)
2 slices ginger root, minced
½ pound asparagus, sliced diagonally
½ cup cashews or cashew pieces
3 scallions, chopped
1½ cups broccoli pieces, cut finely
tamari or soy sauce, to taste
sesame oil for cooking
cooked brown rice

1. Heat wok.
2. Necklace with sesame oil.
3. Stir fry lobster pieces and ginger for 2 to 3 minutes or until lobster pieces are white and firm. Remove to plate.
4. Add asparagus, scallions, cashews, and broccoli to wok. Stir fry till tender (3 to 5 minutes).
5. Return lobster and ginger to wok.
6. Sprinkle with tamari to taste (about 1 to 2 tablespoons) and toss.
7. Serve immediately over brown rice.

SERVES 4

9

SAVORY SOUPS

You can both prepare and serve soups beautifully in your wok.

If you intend to cook a lot of soups in your wok, however, I recommend purchasing a second one, since the constant boiling will eventually wear down the patina.

The following recipes serve 4 with leftovers. These soups are nutritious, delicious, and a great choice for filling yourself up, not *out*!

GARBAGE BAG STOCK

Keeping a plastic garbage bag in your refrigerator is the first step to having a delicious soup stock on hand. It's easy and economical.

Simply save:

Any and all vegetable peelings or trimmings (wash all veggies before peeling)

Our favorites for the most flavor are:

Potato (peels only)
Carrot
Turnip
Onion (also the root end that usually gets tossed out)
Tomato
Cucumber
Sunchoke
Ginger (not too much or it will impart too strong a flavor; but the peelings from 2 to 3 inches of fresh ginger root will give an elusive flavor to a batch of broth)
Garlic
Tough or wilted outer leaves of cabbage or lettuce
Parsley stems
The tough strings from large celery stalks plus trimmings from top and bottom of stalks
Eggshells—yes, eggshells!—well rinsed

Add anything vegetarian you wish to the garbage bag. If you're doubtful about flavor—strength, bitterness, etc.—taste a bit of what you're adding. If the flavor is extremely strong, use your own judgment as to how much of that particular flavor you want in the finished stock. If you end up adding too much of one thing—for instance, ginger peel—you haven't ruined your stock. Simply add another cup of water and taste again. If it is still too stong, cut up 1 small onion, 1 small carrot, add these to the stock, and simmer for another 20 to 30 minutes.

To make stock:

Equal parts "garbage" and water, cup for cup.
Simmer covered 45 minutes to 1 hour.
Strain, cool, refrigerate, or freeze.

This stock can be used for the following "Potage de Garbage" recipe as well as for any other soup base. It can replace water for sauces and even for rice making—it's vitamin packed and tasty as can be.

POTAGE DE GARBAGE

INGREDIENTS:

2 tablespoons oil
½ cup onion, chopped
½ cup carrots, sliced
5 cups garbage bag stock
1 bay leaf
leftover brown rice, bulgur
leftover pasta (if spaghetti, cut into 1-inch pieces)
any leftover cooked vegetables
any leftover cooked meats, diced
leftover mashed potatoes
sea salt to taste
freshly ground pepper to taste
chopped fresh parsley to taste

1. Go through the refrigerator for leftovers. Use one starchy item (rice, bulgur, pasta, potatoes). Any combination of leftover vegetables that suits your fancy will work well. (If you have buttered your vegetables, place the leftovers in a colander and rinse briefly under hottest tap water to remove the butter.) Chicken and shellfish leftovers go well together, as do fish and shellfish. If you have both chicken and fish leftovers, do each of them a favor by using only one of them in your potage. Red meats such as beef, pork, and lamb (if you eat them) may be combined with each other or with chicken, but not with fish or shellfish. If you don't have a starch in your leftover bag and desire a heartier soup, just add a potato or two in step 4.
2. Heat wok over high heat and necklace with oil.
3. Add onion and carrots, and stir fry until onion is translucent and carrots are softened.
4. Add vegetable stock and bay leaf, lower heat, cover, and simmer 20 to 25 minutes until carrots are very tender.
5. Add leftovers you have collected in Step 1. Simmer over medium heat uncovered for several minutes until leftovers are heated through.
6. Add salt and pepper to taste. Ladle into bowls and garnish with fresh chopped parsley.

SERVES 4

SKIP'S "CREAM" OF CARROT SOUP

Here comes Skip again. This time he's invented a "cream" soup for getting skinny on. The trick is *no cream*, just that wonderfully low-calorie tofu! Skip's expertise and originality with food continue to amaze me. Once more, I am most thankful for his invaluable collaboration.

Enjoy his "Cream" of Carrot Soup—guilt-free, of course!

INGREDIENTS:

- 2 tablespoons oil
- 3 cups carrots, scraped and sliced
- 1 tablespoon fresh ginger root, minced
- ½ teaspoon cinnamon
- ½ teaspoon nutmeg
- ¼ cup lemon juice (juice of 1 small lemon)
- 3 cups chicken broth (or water, but broth gives more flavor)
- 2 cups tofu, diced
  sea salt to taste
  freshly ground pepper to taste
- ¼ cup fresh snipped chives (or thinly sliced green tops of scallions)

1. Heat wok over high heat and necklace with oil.
2. Add carrots and ginger root and stir fry 1 minute or until they soften. Do not brown.
3. Add cinnamon, nutmeg, lemon juice, and chicken broth. Bring to boil. Reduce heat, cover, and simmer about 30 minutes until carrots are tender.
4. While carrots are simmering, puree tofu in blender or processor or push through a fine sieve with your fingers or the back of a wooden spoon.
5. When carrots are tender, lift them out of the broth with the strainer and puree them. Return puree to broth.
6. Stir in pureed tofu and blend well over medium heat.
7. Add salt and pepper to taste.
8. Ladle into bowls. Garnish with snipped chives or scallions and serve.

SERVES 4

TAHINI SOUP

INGREDIENTS:

2 tablespoons oil
¼ cup onion, minced
¼ cup celery, minced
⅓ cup brown rice
5 cups boiling water
1 teaspoon sea salt
½ cup tahini (sesame paste)
½ cup cold water
½ cup lemon juice (juice of 2 small lemons)
1 ripe medium tomato, peeled and coarsely chopped*
freshly ground pepper

1. Heat wok over high heat and necklace with oil.
2. Add onion and celery and stir fry until onion is translucent and celery has softened. Do not brown.
3. Add rice. Stir fry briefly to coat rice with oil.
4. Add 5 cups boiling water (which helped you peel the tomato) and salt. Stir once. Cover and reduce heat. Simmer about 40 minutes or until rice is tender.
5. In 1-quart bowl, beat tahini and cold water together until well blended. It will be thick. Add lemon juice and beat until well blended.
6. When rice is tender, ladle off 1 cup of the broth into a measuring cup and beat it by dribbles into the tahini mixture.
7. Stir the tahini mixture into the rice and broth, blending well. Stir in the coarsely chopped tomato. Ladle into soup bowls and sprinkle with freshly ground black pepper.

SERVES 4

* To peel tomato, bring the 5 cups of water to a boil. Spear the tomato through the stem end with a fork and submerge tomato in boiling water for 30 seconds. Skin should peel off easily with a paring knife. If not, return tomato to boiling water for another 10 or 15 seconds and try again.

EGG LEMON SOUP (AVGOLEMONO)

INGREDIENTS:

6 cups chicken broth
½ cup small egg pasta—pastina
2 large eggs
½ cup lemon juice (juice of 2 lemons)
   sea salt to taste
   freshly ground pepper to taste
½ cup scallions, thinly sliced on the diagonal

1. Bring chicken broth to boil in wok.
2. Add pasta. Stir well. Cook according to directions for pasta until pastina is tender.
3. While pastina is cooking, break eggs into medium-size mixing bowl. Beat with whisk or electric mixer until frothy. Add lemon juice and continue beating until mixture is thick and has tripled in volume.
4. When pastina is done, turn off heat and ladle off 1 cup of the broth into a measuring cup. Add the broth by dribbles to the egg/lemon mixture, beating constantly.
5. Stir the egg/lemon/broth mixture into the broth and pasta. Reheat over moderate flame, stirring constantly for 1 minute. Do not simmer or boil, or the eggs will scramble.
6. Add salt and pepper to taste. Ladle into bowls and garnish with sliced scallions.

SERVES 4

AVOCADO YOGURT SOUP

INGREDIENTS:

2 tablespoons oil
1½ cups onion, chopped
½ cup green pepper (sweet or hot or both), chopped
¼ cup celery, chopped
2 tablespoons flour
3 cups chicken broth
½ teaspoon coriander (or to taste)
2 cups avocado cubes
¼ cup lemon or lime juice
1 cup yogurt
hot garnish: crumbled taco chips
cold garnish: chopped tomato

1. Heat wok over high heat and necklace with oil.
2. Add onion, green pepper, and celery. Stir fry until onion is translucent and pepper and celery begin to soften.
3. Stir in flour and blend well.
4. Slowly pour in 1 cup of the broth, stirring well to dissolve flour. Add remaining broth and coriander. Bring to simmer and cook, partially covered, 15 to 20 minutes.
5. Peel, pit, and cube avocado and toss with lemon or lime juice. Puree in batches in blender or processor, or smash with a fork in stainless steel or glass bowl.
6. Puree vegetable/chicken broth mixture and return it to wok.
7. Stir in avocado puree. Reheat just to the simmer.
8. Turn off heat. Stir in yogurt and serve hot or chilled with appropriate garnish.

SERVES 4

POTATO, LEEK, AND SUNCHOKE SOUP

INGREDIENTS:

2 tablespoons oil
2 cups sliced leeks* white part only (or onion or combination of the two), reserving several inches of green
2 tablespoons flour
5½ cups hot water
1 tablespoon sea salt
½ teaspoon white pepper (or to taste)
3¼ cups sliced reserved leek greens
3½ cups boiling potatoes (about 1 pound), peeled and diced
1½ cups sunchokes (Jerusalem artichokes—about ½ pound), peeled and diced
½ cup yogurt (or sour cream or heavy cream if you want to allow yourself a calorie splurge)
3 tablespoons fresh parsley, minced (or dill, especially if you decide to serve this cold)

1. Heat wok over high heat and necklace with oil.
2. Add sliced leek whites (and/or onions) and stir fry over medium heat several minutes without browning.
3. Blend in flour and continue stir frying for 2 minutes to cook the flour. Do not let it brown.
4. Turn off heat. Let mixture cool 1 minute, then gradually stir in 1 cup of hot water. Blend thoroughly, then stir in remaining water.
5. Add salt, white pepper, leek greens, potatoes, and sunchokes. Bring to boil, reduce heat, and simmer gently, partially covered, for 30 to 40 minutes or until vegetables are very tender.
6. Depending on the consistency you want, either leave the vegetables in pieces as they are, mash them in the wok with a potato masher, or, for a truly elegant dish, lift the vegetables out and puree them in a food processor, blender, or food mill. If you choose to puree, return the puree to the liquid in the wok, mix thoroughly, and bring to the simmer again.

* To clean leeks: Trim the white ends off any roots. Cut off all but 3–4 inches of the greens. Slice each leek in half lengthwise. Wash each half under cool running water, making sure to get out all sand that may be lodged between the layers. Shake off excess moisture and proceed as recipe directs.

7. If all the soup will be consumed hot at one meal, you may stir in the yogurt now. Ladle into warm soup bowls and garnish each with a sprinkle of parsley or dill. If you wish to serve leftover soup hot at another meal, simply add 1 or 2 tablespoons of yogurt to each bowl. Yogurt cultures die if they are subjected to high heat. (If you choose to add sour cream instead of yogurt, take the same precaution. Sour cream will curdle if it comes to the boil. If you choose to add cream, you have no problem other than a great increase in calories, since there are no living cultures in sweet cream and it does not curdle when boiled.)

8. Also excellent chilled!

SERVES 4

BEET SOUP

INGREDIENTS:

2 tablespoons oil
2 pounds beets, peeled and grated
½ cup celery, chopped
½ cup onion, chopped
1 cup carrots, shredded
2 cups red cabbage, shredded
4 cups beef broth or water
1 teaspoon sea salt
1 medium potato, peeled and grated

Herb bouquet:

1 bay leaf
4 peppercorns
2 cloves
2 sprigs parsley, wrapped in cheesecloth
sour cream or yogurt for garnish

1. Heat wok over high heat and necklace with oil.
2. Add beets, celery, onion, carrots, and cabbage. Stir fry several minutes until vegetables begin to soften.
3. Add beef broth (or water), sea salt, grated potato, and herb bouquet. Bring to boil. Reduce heat, cover, and simmer gently about 1 hour until vegetables are very tender. Remove herb bouquet.
4. Serve hot or chilled with a spoonful of sour cream or yogurt stirred in each portion.

Note: If you prefer a sweet-sour flavor, add ¼ cup cider vinegar or 1 small lemon, thinly sliced, when you add the broth or water in step 3.

SERVES 4

CHICKEN, MUSSEL, AND SPINACH SOUP

INGREDIENTS:

1 tablespoon oil
2 teaspoons fresh ginger root, minced
½ cup scallions, thinly sliced
1 clove garlic, minced
½ pound boneless chicken breast, julienned
4 cups chicken broth
1 tablespoon tamari or soy sauce
1 tablespoon tahini (sesame paste)
1 pound fresh spinach, washed and trimmed
12–16 mussels, well scrubbed

1. Heat wok over high heat and necklace with oil.
2. Add ginger, scallions, garlic, and chicken. Stir fry for 1 minute.
3. Add chicken broth, tamari, and tahini. Bring to the boil. Lower heat and simmer, covered, for 5 minutes.
4. Add mussels and bring to the simmer. Cover and simmer gently for 8 to 10 minutes or until mussels open.
5. Stir in spinach. Turn off heat. Cover and let steep 1 minute.

SERVES 4

THE KISMET MARKET

Long before the New Yorkers begin their migration to the Fire Island beaches, the natives of these Fire Island communities begin to set up and stock the stores that will service them. I arrived in Kismet in May and spent wonderful days stalking the empty beaches; my evenings were spent sitting in front of roaring fires working on this manuscript without TV, music, or housemates. Sometimes the only diversion I would have all day or week would be my trips to the Kismet Market. Lucky for me, some very special people were to be found there. First there was Paul, an incredibly kind man whose devotion to his work made it possible for me to get the ingredients I needed to work out there. From ginger root to tofu, Paul tried to get it all. Then there's the great lady who works right beside him all summer—his wife, Roz— and their children, Andy, Linda, and Lori. As the summer moves on, smiling new faces appear and soon Daryl, Richard, Craig, Ashley, Loretta, Cathy, Patti, Joey, and Brian came to be a part of the super store without which Kismet could not survive.

By July, when the craziness of too many people and too much partying threatens to drive one insane, the Whitneys and their staff serve as good reminders that August will come and then at last September. Life will become quiet and calm once again and books will actually get finished.

Thank you, friends, for all the warmth all summer long. This one's for you!

BOUILLABAISSE—A MAIN COURSE SOUP

INGREDIENTS:

2 tablespoons oil
1 cup chopped celery (including leaves)
1 cup chopped onion
2 cloves garlic (or to taste), minced
½ cup sliced carrots
1 small bulb fennel, sliced
4 small turnips, sliced
3 tomatoes, chopped
3 cups water, fish stock, or clam juice
2 cups dry white wine
½ teaspoon sea salt (or to taste)
½ teaspoon thyme
  pinch of saffron
¼ teaspoon crushed red pepper
1 bay leaf
2 pounds lean fish fillet cut into chunks (cod, haddock, snapper, perch, sea bass, sea trout, weak fish, flounder, sole, etc. Use all one kind or mix several different kinds.)
1½–2 dozen clams or mussels, well scrubbed
  juice and grated rind of 1 lemon (or more to taste)

1. Heat wok over high heat and necklace with oil.
2. When oil is hot but not smoking, add chopped onion, chopped celery, and minced garlic. Stir fry several minutes until golden.
3. Add sliced carrots, fennel, and turnips, and stir to coat with oil.
4. Add chopped tomatoes, water (or fish stock or clam juice), wine, salt, thyme, saffron, crushed red pepper, and bay leaf. Bring to boil. Simmer over low heat, covered, for about 20 minutes.
5. Add fish pieces, clams, or mussels, lemon juice, and rind. Cover and simmer gently another 15 minutes or until fish is done and clams or mussels have opened.
6. To serve, place several pieces of fish and clams in each bowl, along with some of the vegetables. Ladle hot broth over fish and vegetables.

SERVES 4

MISO

Miso is a dark brown paste usually sold in plastic packets in a health food store. It is very different and certainly worth trying. There are also different types of miso, depending on what the base is made of and the manner of preparation. All of them provide a healthy balance of essential oils, minerals, natural sugars, proteins, and vitamins.

Miso is especially important to vegetarians, since it is one of the few non-meat foods that contains the eight essential amino acids. It has a delicious, unique flavor that makes a great base for soups. A key note with miso is never to boil it, since that destroys some of the essential nutrients.

GARLIC MUSHROOM MISO SOUP

INGREDIENTS:

8–10 dried Chinese or Italian mushrooms
   1 cup hot water
   5 cups vegetable broth
   1 large head garlic, broken into cloves (14–18 cloves)
   1 teaspoon tamari or soy sauce
4–5 drops hot chili oil (or to taste)
   1 cup tofu, diced
   3 tablespoons miso

1. Soak dried mushrooms in 1 cup hot water for 20 minutes or until softened.
2. Bring vegetable broth to boil in wok. Add garlic cloves (unpeeled) and simmer, covered, 20 to 30 minutes until garlic is soft.
3. While broth is simmering, drain mushrooms and rinse them thoroughly (they may be sandy). Remove and discard stems (or save and add to "garbage bag" for next week's vegetable broth). Slice tops thinly and add to simmering broth for final 15 minutes.
4. When garlic is soft and mushrooms have simmered at least 15 minutes, turn off heat and lift out garlic cloves with strainer. You may either discard them or place them in a fine sieve and press the garlic pulp back into the broth. Stir in the tamari, chili oil, and diced tofu.
5. Ladle one cup of the broth into a small bowl containing the miso paste. Blend well and stir into the garlic broth. Cover wok and let mixture steep (without heat) for several minutes. Ladle into bowls and serve.

SERVES **4**

If you get in the habit of making one day a week a "soup-making day," you may find it a hard habit to break.

It's really so easy and such a pleasure to have a jar of soup around!

10

DAZZLING DESSERTS

Treats for you!

Delicious desserts with your best interests at heart.

All of these light, sometimes sugar-free delicacies are show stoppers. The hardest part is getting people to believe you made them in a wok.

But make them in a wok you will—everything from moist cakes to flaming extravaganzas!

Now remember, dessert is a *treat*. A treat is *not* something to have all the time. It's for *special* occasions. Once you are at your ideal weight, begin to play with desserts. Remember, you can cook them a lot, look at them a lot, enjoy their aroma a lot—but *eat just a little!*

JULIE'S KIWI COMPOTE

Ever see the high-fashion jewelry made of gold-dipped feathers? Well, my friend, Julie Waslyn, is responsible for creating them. She's also responsible for creating this next recipe.

Knowing Julie as I do, I was not surprised when her recipe reflected all the color and imagination of a festive occasion. The originality expressed in her jewelry is a reflection of her person, and her recipe follows true to form.

Celebrate with it!

INGREDIENTS:

2 tablespoons unsalted butter
1 large banana, peeled and sliced on diagonal
2 kiwis, peeled and sliced into ¼-inch rounds
1 pint strawberries, hulled and sliced
¼ teaspoon allspice
½ cup freshly squeezed orange juice

1. Melt butter in wok over medium heat.
2. Add banana and stir fry gently and briefly for about 1 minute.
3. Add kiwis and stir fry about 30 minutes.
4. Add strawberries and allspice. Toss gently to combine all ingredients.
5. Add orange juice. Cover wok and turn off heat. Let fruit macerate for 4 to 5 minutes.
6. Serve warm as is or spoon over scoops of vanilla ice cream or slices of pound cake.

SERVES 4

SKIP'S ORANGE COCONUT WOKKED POUND CAKE

INGREDIENTS:

¾ cup (1½ sticks) unsalted butter, softened (or polyunsaturated solid vegetable shortening)

1 cup sugar

3 large eggs, separated

1 teaspoon vanilla extract
grated rind from 1 juice orange

¼ cup freshly squeezed orange juice combined with . . .

¼ cup milk

1½ cups sifted cake flour (not self-rising)

½ teaspoon baking powder

1 cup grated fresh coconut (if you use packaged, look for unsweetened)

⅛ teaspoon cream of tartar
pinch of salt

1. Butter and flour a 6-cup loaf pan (9″ × 5″ × 3″) or round cake pan 9″ × 3″).

2. Sift flour with baking powder and set aside.

3. In 3-quart bowl, cream butter at high speed with electric mixer until light and fluffy.

4. Add sugar gradually, beating constantly until all sugar is incorporated.

5. Separate eggs, one at a time, placing white in a 2-quart bowl and adding yolk to butter mixture. Beat each yolk into butter mixture until well combined.

6. Add vanilla and grated orange rind to butter mixture and beat until well combined.

7. Beating at medium speed, alternately add flour in fourths and orange juice/milk mixture in thirds beginning and ending with flour. Set batter aside.

8. With clean dry beaters, beat egg whites with cream of tartar and salt until they hold stiff peaks.

9. Quickly fold coconut into batter mixture.

10. Quickly but thoroughly fold egg whites into batter so that there are no large clumps of egg whites.

11. Pour batter into prepared pan and place on steamer rack in wok.

Pour boiling water into wok to about ½ inch below steamer rack. Tent with aluminum foil.

12. Place wok cover over aluminum foil and steam cake over medium heat for about 1 hour and 15 minutes. Cake is done when tester inserted in center comes out clean and sides have *just begun* to shrink from sides of pan.

13. Remove from wok. Cool in pan 5 minutes. Turn out on cake rack and cool completely.

SERVES 6

PEACH BREEZE

Named by a man who once delighted New York audiences with his performance in *Grease,* Peach Breeze is Greg Zadikov's favorite, and it really is a breeze to prepare.

INGREDIENTS:

4 cups (about 1½ pounds) fresh peaches, peeled and sliced (or 4 cups frozen, *well drained*)
2 tablespoons lemon juice
1 teaspoon cinnamon
¼ teaspoon nutmeg
¼ teaspoon allspice
2 tablespoons honey
1 cup sifted whole-wheat flour
1 teaspoon baking powder
¼ teaspoon sea salt
½ cup sugar
1 large egg, well beaten
½ cup milk
6 tablespoons unsalted butter, melted
½ cup pecans, chopped

1. Toss peaches with lemon juice, cinnamon, nutmeg, allspice, and honey.
2. Sift flour, baking powder, salt, and sugar together.
3. In 2-quart bowl combine egg, milk, and 5 tablespoons of the butter. Use the remaining butter to grease a 1½-quart casserole or baking dish.
4. Add flour mixture to egg mixture all at once and stir until smooth.
5. Place peaches in buttered baking dish.
6. Pour batter over peaches and sprinkle with pecans.
7. Place on steamer rack in wok. Add boiling water to within ¾ of an inch of rack. Tent with aluminum foil and cover.
8. Steam over medium heat for about 1 hour. Cobbler is done when tester inserted in batter comes out clean. Serve warm or chilled with or without whipped cream.

SERVES 6–8

Note: If you prefer a cobbler with a nicely browned top, remove cobbler from wok when cooked, sprinkle with 2 tablespoons brown sugar, and set under a hot broiler for several minutes until the sugar has melted and is bubbly.

WOKKED AMBROSIA

INGREDIENTS:

2 tablespoons unsalted butter
1 cup fresh grated coconut (or unsweetened packaged)
2 cups fresh grapefruit sections
1 large apple, cored and diced
1 large banana, peeled and sliced
½ cup dates, pitted and sliced
¼ teaspoon allspice
2 tablespoons honey

1. Melt butter in wok over medium heat.
2. Add coconut. Toss to coat with butter and stir fry briskly until coconut is golden and toasted.
3. Add remaining ingredients. Toss to blend well.
4. Cover wok and steam 1 to 2 hours or until heated through.

SERVES 4

SUZANNE LA CROIX' ICE CREAM TEMPURA

This one is a party show stopper.

INGREDIENTS:

1 pint French vanilla ice cream, slightly softened
¼ cup fresh grated coconut
¼ cup toasted cashews, finely chopped

Batter:

1 cup sifted unbleached flour
1 teaspoon baking powder
¼ teaspoon sea salt
1 tablespoon unsalted butter, melted
½ cup water
1 tablespoon lemon juice
1 teaspoon grated lemon rind
2 large eggs
3 cups peanut oil

1. Prepare the ice cream balls in advance. Combine the coconut and cashews on a plate or in a shallow bowl. Line a cookie sheet with waxed paper. With the large end of a melon baller or a tablespoon, scoop and shape ice cream into 1½-inch balls. Roll quickly in coconut mixture and place on cookie sheet. Place in freezer until rock hard. Transfer to airtight container and store in freezer until ready to use.
2. Make batter several hours in advance of serving. Sift flour, baking powder, and salt together in a 2-quart bowl. Beat 1 large egg plus the yolk from the second egg until frothy. Add to dry ingredients along with butter, water, lemon juice, and rind. Stir just until smooth. Beat remaining egg white until stiff and gently fold into batter. Cover bowl and refrigerate for 1 to 2 hours.
3. When ready to serve, heat peanut oil in wok over high heat until oil is very hot (375°F. on deep fry thermometer).
4. Remove ice cream balls from freezer and batter from refrigerator. Dip balls into batter one at a time and drop into hot oil. Deep fry 30 to 45 seconds until batter is golden. Remove from oil and drain on paper towels very briefly (30 seconds or so). Serve immediately.

SERVES 4

SPICED PEARS

INGREDIENTS:

4 large firm ripe pears, halved, cored, and peeled
2 cups dry red wine
1 cup apple juice
½ cup honey
1 bay leaf
8 black peppercorns
4 whole cloves
1 2-inch stick cinnamon
1 1-inch piece vanilla bean

1. Place all ingredients except pears in wok. Bring to boil over high heat and boil uncovered 3 to 4 minutes.
2. Add pears. Reduce heat to medium and simmer uncovered 15 minutes or until pears are tender but not mushy.
3. Carefully remove pears to a large bowl.
4. Over high heat boil liquid remaining in wok until reduced to 2 cups. Strain liquid over pears in bowl. Cool.
5. Serve pear halves with a bit of the liquid spooned over them.

SERVES 4

YUMMY BROWN RICE PUDDING

INGREDIENTS:

- 2 eggs, lightly beaten
- 1 cup apple juice
- ½ cup milk
- 1½ tablespoons honey (or to taste)
- 1 teaspoon vanilla
- 1 teaspoon lemon juice
- ½ teaspoon grated orange peel
- ½ teaspoon cinnamon
- ¼ teaspoon nutmeg
- ⅛ teaspoon salt
- 2 cups plain cooked brown rice
- 1 tablespoon coconut
- ¼ cup raisins or currants
  yogurt or cottage cheese (optional)

1. Mix eggs with apple juice, milk, honey, vanilla, lemon juice, orange peel, coconut, salt, cinnamon and nutmeg.
2. Add raisins or currants and rice. Mix again.
3. Place in slightly oiled baking dish.
4. Place on steam rack in wok over boiling water.
5. Cover and steam 45 minutes.
6. Serve warm or cool with yogurt or cottage cheese.

SERVES **4**

INTEGRAL YOGA INSTITUTE'S CHUNKY APPLE SAUCE

INGREDIENTS:

- 1 ripe banana (in pieces)
- 8–10 apples, sliced in ½-inch chunks
- ½ cup water
- ½ cup raisins
- 1 teaspoon cinnamon (or to taste)
- ¼ teaspoon nutmeg
- 1 tablespoon wheat germ

1. Place apple chunks and banana pieces in wok with water.
2. Cook over low heat till apples start to soften (about 8 to 10 minutes).
3. Add raisins, cinnamon, wheat germ, and nutmeg and stir.
4. Cook 5 more minutes.
5. Serve warm or cold.

SERVES 6

NECTARINE YOGURT FREEZE

INGREDIENTS:

2 cups plain yogurt
¼ cup honey
2 tablespoons freshly squeezed lemon juice
¼ teaspoon cinnamon
⅛ teaspoon nutmeg
¼ teaspoon sea salt
1 pound ripe nectarines, washed, dried, and finely diced

1. Give wok a rest. Use food processor fitted with steel knife, blender, or electric mixer. Combine yogurt, honey, lemon juice, cinnamon, nutmeg, and sea salt in work bowl, blender container, or 2-quart mixing bowl. Process, blend, or beat until well combined.
2. Add finely diced nectarines. Again, process, blend, or beat just until well combined.
3. Pour mixture into an 8-inch square cake pan or into two ice cube trays. Freeze several hours until almost frozen through.
4. Remove from freezer. Cut mixture into small cubes. Place in chilled 2-quart bowl. Beat just until smooth but not melted and runny.
5. Place in 1-quart container. Cover airtight and freeze until firm.
6. Allow to soften slightly before serving to enjoy full flavor of nectarines.

MAKES 1 QT.

CORN PUDDING

INGREDIENTS:

  4 large ears fresh corn (or 2 cups frozen, thawed, and drained)
  1 tablespoon unsulfured molasses stirred into . . .
  ¼ cup honey
  ½ teaspoon cinnamon
  ½ teaspoon mace
  ¼ teaspoon ginger
  ¼ teaspoon sea salt
  2 large eggs, separated
  4 tablespoons unsalted butter, melted

1. Cut kernels from corn cobs. You should have about 2 cups.
2. Puree corn in processor fitted with steel blade or in blender. Add molasses/honey, cinnamon, mace, ginger, sea salt, 2 egg yolks, and 3 tablespoons of the melted butter. Process or blend briefly until mixture is well combined. Pour into 2-quart bowl and set aside.
3. Beat 2 egg whites until stiff but not dry. Fold quickly into corn mixture.
4. With remaining butter, grease a 1-quart casserole or souffle dish. Gently pour corn mixture into buttered casserole.
5. Place casserole on steamer rack in wok. Pour boiling water into wok to within ¾ inch of steamer rack. Tent with foil and cover.
6. Steam over medium heat for approximately 1 hour or until pudding is firm.
7. Serve warm with cinnamon-flavored whipped cream if desired.

SERVES 4

PEARS RICOTTA

INGREDIENTS:

4 very ripe unblemished pears
¼ cup fresh lemon juice
½ cup ricotta
1 tablespoon honey
1 tablespoon golden raisins, chopped
2 dates, pitted and chopped
1 teaspoon crystallized ginger, chopped very fine
⅛ teaspoon ground cloves
2–3 tablespoons toasted slivered almonds

1. Peel pears, slice them in half lengthwise, and remove cores with a melon baller or tablespoon. Dip pear halves in lemon juice to prevent discoloration. Keep halves of the same pear together.
2. Combine ricotta, honey, raisins, dates, ginger, and cloves.
3. Place about 2 tablespoons of the ricotta mixture in a pear half. Cover with 2 pear half. Fill remaining pears.
4. Arrange on individual serving plates and sprinkle with toasted almonds.

SERVES 4

JIMMY GLENN'S BLAZING PINEAPPLE

There is nothing quite like a flaming dessert, so go ahead and impress your friends!

INGREDIENTS:

1 ripe pineapple, peeled, cored, and sliced into thin rounds
¼ cup honey
½ cup water
¼ cup freshly squeezed lime juice
1 cup red currant jelly
½ cup orange-flavored liqueur or brandy
1 cup macaroons, crumbled

1. Combine honey, water, and lime juice in wok. Bring to boil over high heat and add pineapple slices. Reduce heat to medium. Gently simmer pineapple, covered, about 5 minutes or until just tender.
2. Carefully remove pineapple slices from wok and place in warmed serving bowl. Keep warm.
3. Discard all but ¼ cup poaching liquid from wok. Add currant jelly to the reserved liquid and stir over medium heat until melted and hot. Pour over pineapple slices. Sprinkle with macaroon crumbs.
4. Warm liqueur or brandy briefly in the wok. Pour over sauced pineapple.
5. Bring dish to table. Ignite liqueur and carefully spoon Blazing Pineapple into individual serving bowls.

SERVES 4–6

11

MAKING THIS WORK FOR YOU

How and what you eat is a very personal thing. There are ways, though, of making all this work for you.

No matter what your schedule or habits, you can let these new ideas flow into your daily life.

If you work 9 to 5 or if you live alone and find the idea of making dinner every night overwhelming, consider how different and easy this style of cooking really is.

You can cook up a big batch of brown rice once or twice a week and have it in your refrigerator to come home to. That way there will always be something good for you to eat. I live a really busy life myself, so I've gotten into the habit of having rice on hand and merely picking up a fresh vegetable or a piece of fish or simply a breast of chicken on my way home. Stir fried or steamed on stop of the waiting brown rice makes a complete, yet carefree, meal possible in minutes.

Once you get into the habit and feel how easy it really is, then you'll never be *forced* into . . .

... EATING OUT

Eating out is great, *when* you really want to be there. When you're wokking your way skinny and choose to dine out, think Chinese and Japanese. It's much closer to Wokcookery than the fare in American, Italian, or French restaurants. If you're tired of standard Cantonese Chinese, try Szechuan and Mandarin. Though they have the reputation of being hot and spicy, it's not altogether true. Many dishes in these restaurants are not at all spicy.

When you order, it's also a good idea to request the omitting of MSG. MSG is a chemical that expands your taste buds, thereby enhancing the flavor of food. It's a ridiculous notion. Food should be delicious without it, so you don't have to put up with it.

Also, when you're in a restaurant, carry around the same principles that are now a part of your home life. Eat exactly what you want. Don't be intimidated into ordering more. People generally overeat, and restaurants are used to that. If an appetizer is all you want or one dinner to share with a friend, it's your choice. There will always be more food tomorrow. Eat what you really want, and when you're full, *stop.* You don't have to finish what's on your plate. You deserve to treat yourself *carefully* and *delicately,* and by *listening* to *yourself* you will no longer overeat.

Once you start feeling the physical lightness this consciousness produces, you will hate the feeling when you overdo.

That feeling of lightness produces calm, flowing energy and taut, healthy bodies, both of which can change your life.

It opens the door to what I call "unstructured exercise." So even if you've always hated to exercise, with all of this you might find yourself just *moving more,* living a more physical life, and that is the most natural, spontaneous exercise in existence.

Wishing you the body and the life you've always dreamed of—best always,

Annette Annechild

INDEX